BIRTH OVER THIRTY

Sheila Kitzinger, an internationally respected educator and writer, has been exploring different aspects of women's psychosexual experiences for twenty-five years. She brings to her writing a unique ability to translate academic research findings into the kind of practical information women and men can apply to themselves and to their lives.

Born in England and educated at Oxford, she has taught at the University of Edinburgh and done field research on sex, pregnancy, and childbirth among women in settings as diverse as Jamaica, Japan, Mexico, East Germany, and the USSR. She lectures widely in North and South America, Australia, on the continent of Europe, and in Great Britain. In addition to this title, Penguin also publishes *The Experience of Childbirth*, *The Experience of Breastfeeding*, *The Crying Baby*, and *Woman's Experience of Sex*. The mother of five daughters, Sheila Kitzinger lives near Oxford, in England.

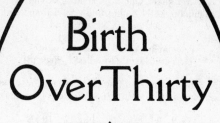

Birth
Over Thirty

—◆—

Sheila Kitzinger
Edited for the United States
by Penny Simkin, R.P.T.

Illustrations by Jo Nesbitt

PENGUIN BOOKS

PENGUIN BOOKS
Published by the Penguin Group
Viking Penguin Inc., 40 West 23rd Street,
New York, New York 10010, U.S.A.
Penguin Books Ltd., 27 Wrights Lane,
London W8 5TZ, England
Penguin Books Australia Ltd, Ringwood,
Victoria, Australia
Penguin Books Canada Ltd, 2801 John Street,
Markham, Ontario, Canada L3R 1B4
Penguin Books (N.Z.) Ltd, 182–190 Wairau Road,
Auckland 10, New Zealand

Penguin Books Ltd, Registered Offices:
Harmondsworth, Middlesex, England

First published in Great Britain by Sheldon Press 1982
This revised and updated edition first published in Penguin Books 1985

7   9   11   13   15   14   12   10   8

LIBRARY OF CONGRESS CATALOGING IN PUBLICATION DATA
Kitzinger, Sheila.
Birth over thirty.
Includes index.
1. Pregnancy in middle age.   2. Childbirth in middle
age.   I. Simkin, Penny, 1938–   .   II. Title.
RG525.K516   1985   618.2   84-1148
ISBN 0 14 02.9997 1

Grateful acknowledgment is made to Olwyn Hughes Literary Agency for
permission to reprint six lines from "Three Women," by Sylvia Plath, from
Winter Trees, copyright © Ted Hughes, 1971, 1972. Published by Faber and
Faber, London, and Harper & Row, New York; and to Professor Gordon
Stirrat and Grant McIntyre Ltd. for permission to quote from Obstetrics.

Printed in the United States of America
Set in Sabon
Designed by Sharen DuGoff Egana

Contents

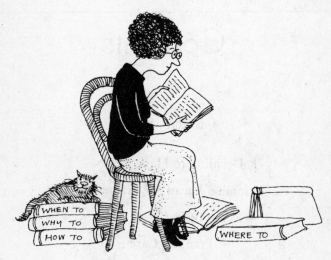

This is not a how-to book

Introduction

More and more women are deciding to have a baby when they are in their thirties or early forties. Yet most books written for expectant mothers imply that they are younger, do not give the specific information an older mother wants, and fail to explore the often complex emotional aspects of birth for a woman who is not merely outside the safest age range in which to have a baby, but who may have a successful career behind her and be in the full activity of creative and rewarding work outside the home.

This is not a how-to book, packed with dos and don'ts. It is based on women's actual experiences and a wide variety of different responses to similar challenges. I am very grateful to all those who wrote about their experiences and have learned a great deal from them. Some of these were people who have been in my own childbirth classes, and I was able to talk with them at length and knew them well. The greatest proportion consisted of 289 women who got in touch following a

Introduction

note in *The Guardian* asking for help. Women in South Africa also started writing following an article in *The Johannesburg Star,* and material from twenty-eight of their letters is included. Women wrote lengthy accounts, often in astonishing detail, and were very open and honest about their negative as well as their positive reactions to the pregnancy, the baby, and the changes that come after the birth.

The gusto with which they wrote was expressed by one woman who, in the middle of her account, suddenly exclaimed: "God, I'm so enjoying writing all this down! It's like a confessional!" As I studied the material I was struck with admiration for women's courage, their capacity for giving, and their strength. Many of the letters were very moving. Some were hilariously funny. The most striking thing was the generous way in which they all shared what they knew. I felt part of a great sisterhood! Sometimes there was a father's account too or a message from older children or from daughters who were themselves late-born children, and these were a bonus.

I have had two children myself while in my thirties, the fourth and fifth in a family of five. But in the book I have concentrated on those aspects of childbirth and parenthood which women themselves talked about most often, rather than approaching it from personal preconceptions concerning what was important. The synopsis with which I started was quite different from the material which eventually emerged.

I have not attempted to include in this book anything about how to prepare for labor. I hope that all older mothers will seek out good childbirth classes, and they

Introduction

may find my book *The Experience of Childbirth* helpful. Nor is there any discussion of practices in specific hospitals or how to choose where to have the baby. That information is in my book *Birth at Home* and is available from local childbirth education groups. Help with the practical and psychological aspects of breastfeeding can be found in *The Experience of Breastfeeding*.

I hope, however, to have written in a way that will mean that the woman over thirty, especially one having her first baby, and the woman over thirty-eight or so having another baby after a long gap, will feel she understands what is happening to her, knows how to take an active part in her pregnancy and birth, and gains in confidence to cope with the challenges before and after the baby comes.

SHEILA KITZINGER
Standlake Manor,
Near Witney,
Oxfordshire

1

Deciding to Have a Baby

Thirty is usually thought of as a watershed in a woman's life, a time for personal stock-taking, but also one full of inherent warnings of failing powers. Before that point she has potential and is a fully sexual being. After it, she is supposed to be past her best and begins to age rapidly. The cosmetics houses, exploiting self-doubts and fears, urge us to buy special "youth dew" and the cream for the "mature" skin with the miracle ingredient guaranteed to plump out degenerating cells.

Women themselves see thirty as a birthday crisis. It is not only that they may look in their mirrors more anxiously for the lines of laughter and experience, but this is a time when they often ask, "Who am I really?" "What am I doing with my life?" "Is this what I want?" and "Where do I go from here?"

The upshot of all this is that more and more women in their thirties and forties are deciding that they will

1

have a baby, either a first baby or another one "before it is too late."

For some, however, it is part of a long-term plan and what they have always intended. Some decide to have a career and *then* babies. Some want babies from early on but discover that circumstances are against them. Claire says she would have had a baby before but could not find the right man and did not contemplate being a single mother. The likely fathers were all "unstable divorcés" who changed their minds when it came to marriage, "leaving me feeling deserted." She did get pregnant "ineptly" by "an immature mature postgraduate," but he did not fancy marriage either, so she went through "the traumatic but fascinating experience of an abortion." When she met a "steady, reliable chap" a year later they married as soon as possible and she became triumphantly, if belatedly, pregnant at thirty-eight.

A late pregnancy may be for very personal reasons because a woman does not feel "ready" before. As one put it:

> I wasn't mature enough to risk having a baby. I needed my work to lose my self-centeredness and be aware of other people's problems. If I'd had a baby earlier I'd have been fighting for my own rights.

Another delayed having a baby because everything she had read about motherhood painted a pretty depressing picture, particularly of "non-working" mothers. "My work was my life for fifteen years. If I had given it up earlier I know I could have resented the baby." Some women embarking on a late pregnancy see it, even then, as, in one woman's words, "a hole in my career for a few years."

Some couples have hoped for a baby for a long time but only get down to doing anything about seeking medical help or starting the more complicated investigations and operations as the thirtieth-birthday crisis looms.

Out of Wedlock

Increasing numbers of women having babies over thirty are not married. Margaret had been frightened of marriage for a long time. She had lived with a man who was violent and destructive and beat her up. When that affair finished, there followed a period in which she could not trust men at all. But then, she said, she realized she was getting "a bit empty inside; all those years of periods and no children." She met a beautiful stranger, did not even know his surname till some months later, and could not speak his language, but knew that she passionately wanted his child. It was partly, she thinks, because she had had to look after elderly parents and their farm for many years and partly because of an inherited Welsh Puritan guilt about enjoying life, that it had all been so delayed. It was a "one-night stand. In *Tess of the d'Urbervilles,* Hardy says that the time for loving and the man to love do not often come at the same time. But for me they did," she says. She conceived that night.

"I don't seem to have a talent for long-term and fulfilling relationships with men," Jane, a writer, explained, "but I don't see why, since I have the great good fortune to be in a position to support my own children, this should stop me being a mother." So she had a very brief encounter with a man when on holiday on a Mediterranean island and, as she put it, was "the classic example of the English spinster abroad throwing her bonnet over the windmill." Even so, when she discovered she was pregnant she was "absolutely terrified" and says her mind was "whirling round like a rat in a trap, moments of heart-stopping terror, and yet these flashes of sheer delight." Another woman in a lesbian relationship says she felt very alone when she saw friends with their children. She was delighted to become pregnant, following artificial insemination, and "now I'm one of the pack!"

There are women living together, too, perhaps in a lesbian partnership, perhaps in a women's commune, who are likely to delay pregnancy until they feel sure this is the right thing to do and that there is enough stability in their relationships for it to be the right time to do it. For these a network of loving women, rather than conventional marriage, offers a basis for embarking on the adventure of bearing and bringing up a child. Some women believe that this may be both a safer and saner environment for a child than one in which male values predominate.

A number of women over thirty who have written to me about why they got pregnant say they did so because they or their husbands were unemployed or laid off, yet one more alarming effect of an economic crisis, with long-term consequences!

4

Deciding to Have a Baby

"Surprise" Babies

Some women conceiving at this age are having "surprise" babies, either totally or half accidentally. A woman concludes, for example, that she has been on the pill long enough, or that she should no longer be on it when over thirty-five, and that it would be safer for her health to use some other method of contraception, and discovers that alternatives are not so reliable. Or she comes off the pill because of its side-effects and decides to "take a chance." Christine stopped the pill because of "debilitating headaches":

> When I eventually realized I was pregnant no one could be more surprised than I. My husband was shocked too, and I felt I had placed a burden on our relationship which took almost five months to untangle. I was terrified at what I had done, but as it was totally my responsibility I came to accept it.

Though she felt guilty about the pregnancy, it does take two to make a baby, and maybe her husband should have been more concerned about her headaches and considered vasectomy. It is, anyway, a classic case of failure of communication between a couple. At least the crisis got them talking to each other again.

Another woman stopped the pill, had amenorrhea (her periods stopped), and was being investigated for infertility:

> I didn't know I was pregnant until I felt the baby move. At first I thought I had indigestion and had been worrying about putting on weight.

5

Birth Over Thirty

This woman is a doctor. She wanted a baby but realizing she was pregnant came as a great shock.

A Roman Catholic who believes it is wrong to use any form of birth control except the "safe period," which she admits was "a laugh," thought it impossible to conceive because her husband had had an operation as a result of which he was told by the surgeons he could not father children. With five children already and very short of money, she felt the pregnancy was a "disaster," and she also felt acutely embarrassed to be pregnant again in her middle forties. But she gradually came to accept "the awful fact," and later, far from hiding the baby in her carriage in the garden, as she thought she would, she "pranced round the village showing her off."

Jane, aged thirty-nine, had taken a year's leave of absence to finish what she calls "a boring academic book" when she discovered she was pregnant. Her first reaction was one of panic, but when she thought about it she says that something in her was "amazed and glad." She was already sharing the house with a close woman friend who was excited by the news and willing to share child care with her. Having made these arrangements her pregnancy was "a long, dreamy, and tranquil time." The coming baby was like a gift, arriving at what she was aware was near the end of her reproductive life. She felt not only special, but blessed, and she describes it as "the Saint Elizabeth syndrome," though other people were telling her that she must be mad and her own mother was "shocked and upset," accusing her of irresponsibility and saying that she only hoped her child would never cause her the sorrow that she had brought to her mother. She found the whole experience of pregnancy and childbirth, even a very painful and difficult labor, a deeply satisfying one.

Decisions, Decisions

Even when conception is an accident the decision to go ahead with the pregnancy is usually a conscious and carefully thought out one, and there is no mistake about that. Women often feel under pressure all the same and, like Christine, are submerged under waves of guilt. One woman said she was under open pressure from her anxious psychiatrist advising her to have an abortion when she became pregnant during a serious depressive illness. She found this terribly upsetting, partly because she was feeling very pleased with herself for the first time in years. She continued with the pregnancy, feeling guilty but "secretly rather smug" and "one up" on the psychiatrist. By the time the baby was five months old she no longer needed a psychiatrist.

Feeling guilty can mean that a pregnancy continues because the alternative seems too awful. Harriet, aged forty, went to the hospital to have an abortion, where the nurse preparing her for the operation said, "Whatever will sister say?" Then sister came in, shook her head, and remarked, "Oh dear, doctor won't like *this!*" Harriet got up and left. Whatever the doctor thought, it was she who was having the baby and who was committed to bringing up the child afterward. Pressures can also be exerted the other way and a late pregnancy be made to sound like an ominous and nasty illness, bearing such great risks of having an abnormal baby that a woman feels she cannot go through with it for this reason alone.

The single mother may have special qualms about the decision she has taken. One said that all through pregnancy she kept wondering whether she was doing the right thing in planning to keep the baby, but felt sure she wanted it with a more consistent longing than she ever had for a man. "Lynne Reid Banks [a contemporary British novelist] has that rather corny bit about the love for the child being like a steady flame whereas sexual love flickers on and off," she added.

Occasionally a pregnancy catches the woman in her forties so much by surprise that, thinking she is beginning the menopause, she does not find out she is pregnant until it is too late for an abortion. This happened in a distressing way with Elizabeth, after a brief temporary reconciliation with her former husband when she was recovering from alcoholism. One day she felt flickering movements in her abdomen and it dawned on her with horror that she was pregnant. She felt she owed it to the baby to give her up for adoption, but found it very difficult in the home for unmarried mothers, where most of the women, who were all much younger, intended to keep their babies. One girl told her, "You treat it like it was throwing away dirt."

But most women having babies at this age do so because this is what they want. And even if the decision is one that follows on the fact of conception, the realization brings not only shock and some apprehension, but a delighted surprise and bubbling, if submerged, excitement.

There are also, of course, second marriages, second

Deciding to Have a Baby

"chances" in life, bringing with them second, or sometimes first-off, families, or at least "one for him." With any woman who already has grown-up or school-age children, the decision-making is mixed with anxiety about how the older ones will cope. Will they see it as a loss of love? Can they handle the experience of having new family members younger than them as well as a new proxy father? What effect will a baby sibling have on adolescents who are still very uncertain of their own sexuality and their own identity? Perhaps they will never come home; perhaps they will feel that mother is somehow competing with them; perhaps they will feel rejected and unwanted.

Some of those who have babies at this age have been happy and confident in their careers and only feel able to go ahead and have a baby when they feel satisfied they have achieved something in their working lives. Motherhood then comes as a welcome fresh start and something else in which they hope they can also use their skills.

One woman who wrote had already decided on sterilization. Her lover mentioned having children, but she says she ignored this and assumed the remarks "were just sentimental indulgences brought on by a new relationship." Arrangements for the operation were delayed because she was going on holiday and then she had a conference to attend. During this time she began to feel that having a baby with this particular partner would be "a shared affair, and not me as a female founding a dynasty for some man." She went ahead and had a child, though the couple do not live together and do not intend to in the future. The plan is for the baby to be in her mother's home for the first two months, with her father there for most of the time too, and then for the baby to move to the father's apartment.

New Responsibilities

For some women it comes as a shock that the confidence they felt in teaching or running a business, for example, wanes when they are faced with the responsibilities of caring for a baby and they have to come to terms with themselves in a new way.

Delia, aged forty-two, had been a very capable social worker accustomed to dealing with confused adolescents, distressed mothers, social derelicts, and senile old people. She was amazed at her vulnerability and the swing of her constantly changing emotions in the hospital after having the baby: "How *could* I have let them boss me around like that? And why did I get so worked up about the different advice coming from all and sundry?" And when she went on feeling utterly incompetent and dogged with anxiety throughout the first year after the baby's arrival she realized that she was suffering from chronic postnatal depression. She needed to talk about it and to be able to get on the telephone to someone supportive when she felt most isolated. When she was able to do this, she worked through the experience and believed that she had learned something about herself. She is not the invincible, all-giving person as whom she had masqueraded. There are times when she needs to *take* as well as to give, and she can now relax and receive from other people as well.

Deciding to Have a Baby

Other women start out on motherhood at this age largely because they feel they have never succeeded completely at anything else and hope that this is something they can do at last. Though it might seem they would be doomed to failure and that it is one of the worst reasons for having a baby, nearly all those who have described to me this emotional journey feel they have discovered themselves and have a new maturity and security. Perhaps it was when they began to trust themselves and have the courage to make decisions based on their own experience of life that the step was already taken, and the pregnancy confirmed this rather than being the cause of it.

Sue, for example, said she was a "failed academic." She had always felt slightly apologetic about her job as a nursery school teacher with her first partner, himself an academic. They had a baby but she felt torn between her work and looking after the child, and guilty about her part-time mothering. They were unhappy together and the relationship broke up. Four years ago, when her daughter was six, she started to live with Dan, another academic. She gave up work outside the home when they had a baby, and, in spite of feeling diminished in status by being "only a mother" when with feminist friends who have put mothering gladly behind them or never taken it on, admits that having a baby "releases" her to "putter about with justification," something she has always wanted to do but has never had the confidence to admit. Perhaps one of the most important things for Sue is that she does not feel alone in caring for the baby, as if it is a task only she could do and for which innate "maternal instincts" are

11

sufficient. Dan shares in everything, including the night work, and is almost as involved as she is herself. Because he does not feel it is second-class work, she is not put on the defensive about her role as a mother.

Reason to Conceive

Some babies are conceived nowadays because the woman wants satisfying work outside the home and, in the present economic situation, cannot get it. Frustrated in the need for a job which meets her abilities, she opts for a baby almost as a second-best choice. This may work in the early days, but once the child is at school she is faced with the problem again. There are added financial responsibilities, and she has renewed ties at home. The baby has allowed her to bridge a difficult time, but the same difficulty reasserts itself.

One reason why a couple may put off having a baby is that one or the other partner, or both, have come from an unhappy family and do not want to perpetuate this misery. One woman told me, for example, "My own family has given me a poor pattern of personal relationships, and I felt trapped in my parents' failure." This kind of impediment in the emotional background can mean that neither partner is certain about whether it is right to have a baby at all. One partner usually gains in confidence through the other's love over the years, and the sense that now is the time to start out on the adventure of parenthood together grows out of the feeling of satisfaction in the couple's relationship. Without it, neither may ever feel ready for a child. Janet delayed till she was nearly forty for this reason but is now "hooked" on having babies. "I am," she said, "like a convert to a new religion!"

Some women admit they had a baby, or another baby, for selfish reasons. "If I had heard anyone else give this reason," Geraldine confessed, "I would have thought they were mad. It was quite irrational. I was very depressed, hated the house we live in, resented doing anything to it or buying anything for it." Her three children were at school and her husband immersed in his civil-service career, caught up in "the rat race." "I wanted to tie myself down to the family again. I knew I was drifting away and thought I could recapture some of the happiness we had earlier in our marriage." One can imagine what some marriage counselors might say about such motives for starting a baby. Babies cannot really be used to patch a failing relationship, or, at least, if they are conceived in this hope, other things have to happen between the couple before any fresh start can take place. Fortunately Geraldine and David both responded to the challenge, and after a frightening first year or so following the birth, when she was depressed and felt she was living under a permanent black cloud, they talked things through as they never had done before and made radical adjustments in their life together. He gave up his job, which was a demanding one and meant that he really saw the children only on weekends, and took another which allowed Geraldine to do a postgraduate degree and him to look after the family for one day a week, as well as share much more in caring for all four generally. She at last feels a person again and says she has learned, "It is too easy to become a passive dependent." She had believed herself indispensable in this passive role, but now realizes that "there's nothing I do for my children that they cannot either do for themselves or that someone else can do for them." This is "liberating knowledge" and gives her freedom to enjoy them as people rather than objects to be serviced. The stress of having a baby in an unhappy relationship such as this one was can be used constructively to push the couple out of a rut, but they have to be able to make use of the experience and to *create* change, not just let things happen to them.

New Dependency

For a woman who has been busily occupied with her career however, pregnancy brings with it a new dependency in which she may luxuriate and enjoy the sense of being cherished. Sally had a demanding job in public relations and says that children were just "things that happened to friends." Her first marriage broke up and she remarried and started a family at thirty-five: "I loved being treated in a special way by everyone." This feeling of being valued has continued after the births of her two children largely because her husband is a "sharing, caring partner in all things." For other women the sense of worth gained by the pregnancy is readily destroyed when caring for a new baby in social isolation. They soon feel drained of strength, and of their selfhood.

Another woman who welcomed being "taken over" by a process she trusted completely said she had had "jolly good innings" in her professional career, "twenty years of freedom to plan my own life and spend time on what appealed to me," and now pregnancy and birth brought for the first time "something taken out of my hands . . . to use me." She enjoyed being in touch with her feelings in a new way and the sense that life was expressing itself *through* her, while she learned the flexibility to respond to its demands.

Many women say that pregnancy also brings a sense of oneness with creation, even though they may never have thought of themselves as religious or mystical. The feeling of nurturing another life, of being part of a universal tradition, was how one woman described her exultation in pregnancy.

Being with child also changes other people's ideas of you. "Male colleagues at work," one woman says, "seem to see me in a different role. (Perhaps I'm not so threatening now!) They beam at me all the time with stars in their eyes and talk about their children." She enjoyed seeing this different reflection of self in those with whom she was in constant contact.

We do not usually put such pleasures into words, and perhaps they sound minor when we do, but for anyone, a woman or a man, who has been scurrying around issuing documents and posting bits of paper to other people who are engrossed in the same activities, life when a baby is on the way and as a parent takes on a completely new meaning.

This is what seems to have happened for Shelley, who had been a *Playboy* bunny and then an airline hostess. When she married a man much older than herself she had her IUD taken out and conceived immediately. There had been no time to consciously think about the effects on their relationship or why she was trying to get pregnant. But looking back at it now she says:

> Without a doubt if Josh had not come we would have been divorced. To me our marriage would have been like a long date and I would have packed him in as I had done with many previous boyfriends. What a blessing I hung in there because now I realize what a wonderful soul mate I have, and my happiness often frightens me.

There is another passive acceptance of pregnancy however, which has a more negative aspect. This is the mental state in which a woman considers termination because she really does not want the child but cannot face the abortion. Ann said she was frightened and deeply shocked when she learned she was pregnant at forty-one. She went to an abortion clinic, but was too confused and uncertain to go through with the operation. For several weeks after she refused to acknowledge that she was pregnant, but "when I had to accept it I was plunged into deep depression, sitting for long periods in a large armchair like a hamster in a nest." The inner anger she felt continued throughout the pregnancy, but once she started her prenatal care and someone else obviously cared about the baby, she began to feel she could cope. In a way she handed over her emotional link with the baby. Fortunately she and her husband could afford day care and she was soon back at work. Now fifty-five, she says, "My husband delights in her. As for me—well, I love her but at times I wish there was no child at home." It sounds as if both Ann and her daughter are missing out, but perhaps there was no other way.

A Painful Longing

A woman may come off the pill when she has been on it for many years, or give up her job intending to settle down to a pregnancy at last, only to discover that she is subfertile and that it is difficult to start a pregnancy, or to hold on to one that has started. This is sometimes the reason why a baby is delayed into the forties, and there has been a lengthy period of tests and investigations preceding the successful pregnancy. The longing for a baby becomes a painful daily reality, with each period like a miscarriage, and the couple are under the continual stress of working out ovulation and the right moment for intercourse in spite of their own spontaneous feelings. The burden may become so intolerable that the relationship itself is subjected to strain. Sometimes a period is delayed just long enough for the woman to feel that this time, surely, it must be, but then she experiences the all-too-familiar sensations of the beginning of menstruation.

Susan gave up her job when she was thirty-five, a year after she was married, to improve her chances of conception. Two years later she had a call from her GP to tell her that her pregnancy test was positive, but she lost the baby within the next few hours. This was followed by a phantom pregnancy in which she had many of the signs of pregnancy, including cessation of periods, abdominal swelling, nausea and vomiting, and what she mistakenly thought were fetal movements. It was a psychological trick in which her body acted out her passionate desire for a child. As a result she was very skeptical about any possible pregnancy after that and, when her fortieth birthday came, decided firmly that she was giving up any idea of pregnancy and went on a twenty-four-mile walk. She conceived the next day. She felt as if in physically walking the notion of having a baby out of her system she had freed her body to become pregnant.

For many couples getting pregnant seems to be simpler when they are on holiday and away from their ordinary day-to-day routines. Victoria and Tom were on a Greek island with other couples who had small children: "two adorable little girls at what Tom calls the 'Mary Janes and pinafores stage.' He got rather broody and under the influence of relaxing sunshine, the holiday sun, and the odd bottle of retsina, I said, 'Why don't we have another one or two before I'm too old?'" Another couple was on holiday in Portugal, where she lost her packet of contraceptive pills. They decided not to try to get hold of any more. Two others were white-water canoeing, and during the long dark evenings, when there was nothing else to do, made love, came to the conclusion that they would like to have a baby, and made love again!

Reading all this you may feel that none of these women are like you and that your motives for having a baby after thirty are different and perhaps more complex. However it is, it can be helpful to ask yourself, why do I want this baby? This is not because you can produce a snap answer or know exactly why you do, but because increased self-awareness, including understanding of those aspects of ourselves which are least salutary, might enable us to be better mothers and more psychologically rounded human beings.

2

Planning Ahead for Pregnancy

Planning ahead for pregnancy is usually part of the scheme for women having their first babies over thirty and for a good many of those having a late baby. They have often used contraception for a prolonged period, sometimes since their teens, and make a conscious decision to stop and get pregnant.

A word of warning here, though. Do not just come off the pill and hope to get pregnant. Use another method of contraception (a condom, for example) for three months so that there is little chance of hormones from the pill remaining in your bloodstream when you conceive. Oral contraceptives have a systemic effect. Every cell in your body is affected. You need to leave time for it to get back to normal. Artificial progesterone, on which the mini-pill, one of the most commonly prescribed contraceptive pills, is based, can cause masculinization of a female fetus if taken during pregnancy.[1] The incidence of miscarriage and birth defects is also increased.[2]

Planning Ahead for Pregnancy

The Pill and Your Diet

Oral contraceptives reduce the absorption of vitamins of the B group. When looking ahead to pregnancy, check your diet to make sure that you are getting a large amount of foods containing these vitamins. They include liver, herring, and salmon; brown rice, walnuts, peanuts, wheat germ, and whole-wheat products (such as bread and breakfast cereals); yeast and black molasses. It may be better to avoid liver, however, since animals are sometimes fed estrogens to plump them up, and this means that you are inadvertently absorbing more hormones with meat.

Pill users also have a reduced uptake of vitamin C. This in turn may reduce iron absorption and interfere with synthesis of some natural hormones. The best source of vitamin C is fresh fruit, raw vegetables, and baked potatoes in their jackets. A large glass of fresh orange juice (rather than canned or frozen) every day will ensure a good basic level. All green vegetables, including parsley, broccoli and sprouts, and sweet peppers are rich in vitamin C. Citrus fruits are particularly good sources.

Occasionally folic acid is low in pill users. Alcoholic drinks lower its absorption still further. Low levels of folic acid have been implicated as possibly causing some birth defects, including spina bifida. Include in your daily diet some foods rich in folic acid: asparagus, spinach, bran, whole-wheat bread and cereals, dried beans of any kind, yeast. Folic acid is present in liver, too, but again you may wish to avoid it. Low levels of zinc can be met by drinking a glass of milk every day, since zinc is added to cattle food. Zinc is also present in freshly picked vegetables, especially peas, and in whole-wheat breads and cereals. Use as little cooking water as possible when preparing vegetables (it conserves the flavor better anyway). Then save the cooking water for soup stock when you can. Some pill users are also short of another trace element, magnesium. This is found in milk, nuts, and whole-grain products, too.

It is rarely necessary or desirable to take vitamin pills, popular though these are, especially in the United States, where even a "pill pill" has been produced to counter the effects of the contraceptive pill. Excess amounts of vitamins and minerals, especially those which are stored in the body such as A and D, can do more harm than good. Above all, avoid vitamin A supplements after being on the pill, since excess of this vitamin may be associated with birth defects and vitamin A levels are raised by 30 to 80 percent in women taking the pill. Levels of A take up to three months to return to normal. For this and other material on side effects of the contraceptive pill which may be relevant to pregnancy, see *Women and the Crisis in Sex Hormones,* by Barbara and Gideon Seaman (New York: Bantam, 1978). A nutritious and balanced diet every day is the best protection against vitamin deprivation.

Coming Off the Pill

Though some studies have suggested that being on the pill for years reduces fertility, recent research shows that the great majority of women wanting to get pregnant after years on it conceive without difficulty. Perhaps those who do not have always been infertile but did not know it. Occasionally, too, a woman in her early forties does not get pregnant because she is having an early menopause and there are no more follicles inside her ovaries to ripen. If you come off the pill and normal menstruation does not return, check that you are having adequate nutrition in terms of calories. Undernutrition has been shown to reduce fertility. It is a major cause of amenorrhea and failure to ovulate. On the other hand, some women may be slow to rid their bodies of hormones in the pill and be infertile for a year or so after. Some do not menstruate during this time. But even if you menstruate, it does not necessarily mean that you are ovulating regularly.

If after three months off the pill you have started regular periods and notice that your breasts swell at that time, you can take it for granted that you are ovulating. If you are aware of some premenstrual tension, so much the better!

If you have had an IUD and it is removed prior to pregnancy, you may possibly be anemic, since anemia from menstrual heavy bleeding is five times more common among women with an intrauterine device than those using other contraceptive methods.[3] If you have a history of heavy bleeding, whether or not you have had an IUD, iron supplements may be in order before you start a pregnancy. Your doctor will be able to tell you this after doing a simple blood test. Do not leave iron therapy until after you become pregnant.

Folic Acid

There is one situation in which taking a multivitamin pill which contains folic acid too may be advisable, whether or not you have been taking oral contraceptives. This is when you or someone closely related has previously had a pregnancy in which the fetus had an abnormality of the central nervous system—spina bifida or anencephaly. A woman who has had a baby with a central nervous system defect has ten times the chance of having another baby similarly affected. Research in Liverpool[4] and in Wales,[5] both areas in which there is a high rate of these handicaps, with women who already had babies who suffered from these abnormalities or had pregnancies terminated because the fetus was deformed, suggests that taking extra vitamins and folic acid in capsule form for three months *before* conception and during the first two or three months of pregnancy dramatically reduces the recurrence rate of these conditions. There is some argument as to whether vitamins or folic acid help most and, if it is vitamins, which ones are important, so though you may feel that you are taking a mackerel to catch a sprat, it is worth having capsules which contain vitamins A and D, thiamine, riboflavin, pyridoxine, nicotinamide, ascorbic acid, folic acid, ferrous sulphate, and calcium phosphate. The usual dose is one capsule or tablet three times a day. There is no value in taking more than that. Further research into folic acid is taking place, complicated by the fact that in some animals extremely *high* levels of folic acid are also associated with fetal deformities.

If you want to terminate a pregnancy with an abnormal fetus, make certain that you get AFP (see pages 48–49) testing, and if levels of AFP are high, go on from there to have amniocentesis at the end of the fourth month of pregnancy (see Chapter 3). This kind of forward planning can do a lot to lower levels of anxiety through pregnancy.

Smoking

If you smoke, even if it is only occasionally or a few a day, stop well before you become pregnant. Smoking increases the risk of miscarriage, premature birth, and a small-for-dates baby (one who is not up to the anticipated size for that particular week of gestation) as a result of a poorly functioning placenta: the flow of blood is reduced on the mother's side of the placenta, and that blood is short of oxygen. Once the oxygen reaches the baby, it cannot flow easily through the baby's circulatory system because blood vessels have become constricted and the blood itself is stickier than normal.[6] When a pregnant woman lights up, her baby's heartbeat speeds up, and recent research shows that for a smoker even to *think* about having a cigarette has an effect on the fetal heart.

The fetus makes breathing movements in preparation for breathing after birth. When the mother is smoking, the amount of oxygen is reduced, these movements cease to be rhythmic, and the fetus seems to be literally gasping. There may be long-term effects on the child. At the age of seven the children of women who smoked during pregnancy are slightly behind others in reading and some other skills. There is only one advantage to smoking in pregnancy, and that is a doubtful one: a smoking mother is less likely to develop pre-eclampsia. This is a disease peculiar to pregnancy, the symptoms of which are raised blood pressure, albumin (protein) in the urine, and fluid retention. If she *does* get it, she gets it worse than a nonsmoking mother, and the outcome for the fetus is worse.[7]

The baby's father should also stop smoking before conception. German research suggests that chemical poisons in tobacco may produce abnormal sperm.[8] You also should not have to breathe in a smoke-laden atmosphere. This is known as "passive smoking," and there is disagreement about its dangers. But if there is any chance that it could interfere with a baby's health, many mothers would try to avoid inhaling other people's tobacco smoke. Unfortunately it is not considered polite or sporting to ask friends and work colleagues to stub out their cigarettes, and it can be embarrassing when you are still in early pregnancy and have not yet told them about it. But some expectant mothers feel forced to do this anyway because the smell of cigarettes makes them feel nauseous. Even if you smoked before, you may be revolted by it in the first three months of pregnancy and can feel trapped in a restaurant, for example, when others at the table light up. Of course you can always lean over your acquaintance's meal and say, "I'm pregnant and smoking makes me vomit."

Though smoking reduces a baby's birth weight by 3 to 6 ounces, fortunately middle-class women who smoke often have good-sized babies. It is the baby at risk for some other reason, too, who has another condition which interferes with growth in utero, for ex-

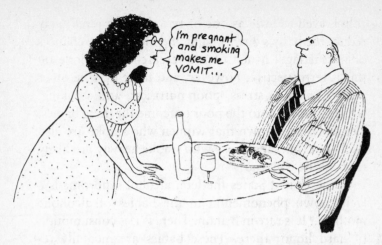

ample, or who is indirectly the victim of social conditions in which its mother has to live, who is most likely to suffer from the effects of maternal smoking. Some women are so addicted to smoking that they cannot give it up without causing severe stress. If you have a choice, however, avoid cigarettes for your baby's sake.

Some women who give up smoking in early pregnancy start again when they are waiting for the results of amniocentesis (see Chapter 3). Others who smoke lightly find themselves smoking more heavily under the stress of waiting to know whether the baby is all right. If you are aware of this in advance you may be less willing to light the first cigarette.

Alcohol

Heavy alcohol consumption is hazardous for the baby. But it has now been discovered that some women cannot safely drink any alcohol at all in pregnancy. Alcohol, even as little as one or two drinks a week, may reduce the baby's birth weight and increase the chances of miscarriage. Much of the research being done on this is retrospective, however, and there may be other factors, such as stress, poor nutrition, and smoking, which contribute to the poor outcome for these babies. Certainly it is known that women who smoke are also likely to drink, and those who smoke heavily are likely to drink heavily too.

In the United States the fetal alcohol syndrome is a well-known phenomenon in the babies of alcoholic mothers.[9] It is rare in Britain. There is less consumption of hard liquor there. These babies are mentally retarded, growth-retarded, and tend to have central nervous system abnormalities and heart problems. They have a characteristic facial appearance with a rather heavy jaw and flattened bridge of the nose.

Though the fetus is vulnerable at any stage of pregnancy, the periods when alcohol most affects brain growth are weeks twelve to eighteen and weeks twenty-four to thirty-six. It is worth thinking through your attitude to alcohol before you become pregnant and deciding what you want to do.[10]

Drugs

Though some drugs are known to have a teratogenic effect (producing congenital malformations) and should never be taken if you are intending to get pregnant, there are a great many others about which little is known. They may be absolutely harmless or, depending on when they are taken and the dosage, one baby in several

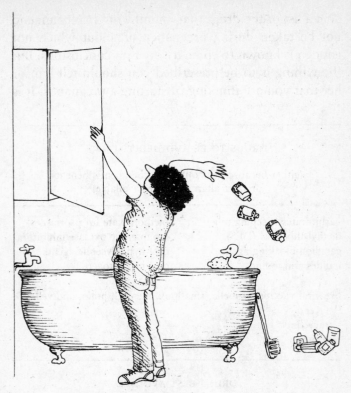

Throw out anything in the bathroom cupboard which has been prescribed before

thousand or fifty thousand or a hundred thousand is affected by them. This is why it is best to avoid all drugs, even over-the-counter household medications like aspirin and indigestion tablets, if you are planning on getting pregnant. In practice this is not always possible, and it is then necessary to weigh the benefits and disadvantages of taking a particular drug. Your physician or midwife can help you with this and will have available a list of the drugs that manufacturers recommend not be taken during pregnancy or about which not enough is known to come to any firm conclusions. But if anything is to be prescribed you should tell him or her that you are thinking of starting a pregnancy. It is

---

DRUGS TO BE AVOIDED TOTALLY

(either because risks outweigh therapeutic benefits
or safer alternatives are available)

---

barbiturates (sleeping pills)	methotrexate for psoriasis
diethylstilbestrol (DES)	monoamine oxidase inhibitors
ganglion-blocking agents	oral hypoglycemic agents
iodides and iodine	oral progestogens

live viral vaccines (rubella, smallpox, measles, polio, and yellow
 fever)
tetracycline
reserpine

DRUGS BEST AVOIDED

In First Trimester	Throughout Pregnancy
antacids	co-trimoxaole
iron supplements	diazoxide
metronidazole	ergotamine
salicylates (aspirin)	hypnotics
	propranolol
	sulfa drugs
	lithium carbonate
	prostaglandin synthetase inhib- itors
	thiazide diuretics (water pills)

DRUGS TO BE USED
UNDER SPECIALIST SUPERVISION

(and only when essential)

aminoglycoside antibiotics
anticoagulants (to reduce
    blood clotting)
antithyroid drugs
chlorpromazine
diazepam
chlordiazepoxide
chloroquine

cytotoxic drugs
hypotensive agents (to lower
    blood pressure)
lithium carbonate (in mental
    illness)
systemic corticosteroids (for
    asthma)

also wise to throw out anything in the bathroom cupboard which has been prescribed before. If you are away from home and get ill, even if it is just a bout of holiday diarrhea, tell the doctor that you think you may be pregnant and ask whether the prescription is safe for early pregnancy. This is one of the things that ought to be added to foreign-language phrase books!

The first three months of pregnancy are those when the fetus is most vulnerable, since it is then that the main structures of the body are being formed. At two and a half months the placenta starts functioning. It is often described as a filter, but in fact it is a sieve which allows through many drugs, depending on their molecular size.

Barbiturates cross the placenta rapidly, can alter the baby's fluid balance, may cause goiter, and, if taken at the end of pregnancy, can interfere with the baby's breathing at birth. They should be avoided in pregnancy. DES (diethylstilbestrol) is the notorious drug which causes a special kind of cancer of the vagina of some daughters of women who have taken it at the beginning of pregnancy. It was used in an attempt to avoid miscarriages, but was ineffective at this anyway. Iodides are used for the treatment of thyroid conditions; they cross the placenta and can cause hyperthyroidism (overactivity of the thyroid gland) and goiter (enlargement of the gland) in the baby. Some cough medicines contain large quantities of iodides.

Vaccines

Live viral vaccines may infect the baby. Rubella (German measles) vaccine is of this kind. Check with your doctor to be sure you are immune. If you need immunizing, postpone pregnancy for three months afterward.

Children immunized against polio with oral vaccine excrete the virus and very rarely affect their mothers. If you have never been immunized against polio you should be immunized at the same time as your child, but first make sure that you are not already pregnant.

Monoamine oxidase inhibitors are psychotropic drugs from which a woman needs to be weaned gradually, best of all before she becomes pregnant, but if not, soon afterward.

If you are diabetic and hoping to have a baby, discuss this with your specialist before you get pregnant. Reserpine, used to lower blood pressure, should not be used in pregnancy as it may slow down the heart rate of the fetus, interfere with the baby's temperature control after birth, and make it drowsy at delivery. Babies of mothers who have been on reserpine may also get swelling of the mucous membrane in their noses so that they cannot breathe. Tetracycline, an antibiotic, is on the list of drugs to be avoided because it can cause a yellow stain on the baby's first teeth and may slow down bone growth. The sulfa drugs, which are used to treat bacterial infections such as cystitis and streptococcal infections, interfere with folic acid synthesis, though they have been used for many years.

Some people think that the more iron you can get, the better. This is not true, because taking iron pills unnecessarily can produce hemoglobin cells which are so large that they will not pass through the finer blood vessels in the baby, who is then deprived of some of the oxygen-carrying blood which would otherwise reach it. The routine administration of iron supplements in pregnancy seems unwise and often causes nausea in the first few months and constipation right through pregnancy. Find out if you are anemic before taking any extra iron.

Aspirin

Aspirin interferes with blood clotting and is suspected of causing birth defects if taken in large doses in the first few weeks of pregnancy. Because it affects blood clotting, if a large amount is taken in the last week before the baby is born it could cause hemorrhage in the newborn.

Sulfa drugs, used for the treatment of urinary infections, inhibit folic acid metabolism. They should definitely not be taken in the first weeks, and since their safety has not been proved, it is best to avoid them throughout pregnancy. Ergotamine is present in migraine medicines. Since it may cause the uterus to contract, migraine should be treated with alternative drugs and preferably with rest in a darkened room before the symptoms have time to build up.

Sleep medications cross the placenta and are best avoided because they dope the baby along with the mother. Propranolol is used for heart disease, but also crosses the placenta and can affect the baby's heart. Sometimes it has to be used, but then only for cardiac disease, not for high blood pressure. Thiazide diuretics used to be very fashionable in pregnancy to reduce water retention, especially in the United States, where they were combined with strict dieting to limit weight gain in pregnancy. This is very dangerous.

Several drugs are known to cause damage to the baby's retina when used in high doses. One is chloroquine, used to treat malaria. Another is chlorpromazine, used in the treatment of mental illness, but no damage has been observed with low doses. Diazepam (Valium) crosses the placenta and can cause respiratory depression in the baby, poor muscle tone and feeding problems. Chlordiazepoxide (Librium) does too. (These three drugs may have to be used occasionally, nevertheless.) Lithium carbonate crosses the placenta, can alter the fetal fluid balance and cause goiter.

Warfarin is an anticoagulant which crosses the placenta and if used earlier in pregnancy should be replaced by heparin four weeks before the baby is due, since it stops the baby's blood clotting. Heparin, how-

ever, does not cross the placenta. Steroids sometimes
have to be used in pregnancy for severe asthma, but if
alternative therapy works it should be used, as there is
evidence of extra risk to the baby. Local and regional
anesthetics cross the placenta too. If you have to have
an anesthetic for anything in early pregnancy, let the
doctor or dentist know that you think you may be
pregnant.

X Rays

Most people are wary of X rays and realize that they
are cancer-inducing. If there is any possibility that you
might be pregnant or plan to get pregnant before your
next period is due, avoid an X ray of the abdomen,
pelvis, or lower back. The risk to the baby is highest
in the first twelve weeks of pregnancy, and if the fetus
is exposed to twenty-five rads or more during this time
termination is advisable. Some people suggest that pelvic X rays, if considered necessary, should be done only
in the first half of a woman's menstrual cycle in case
she becomes pregnant, but the ovum may be affected
whether it is the first or second half. After the twelfth
week of pregnancy it has been estimated that the highest risk to the baby of developing leukemia is in the
order of 1 in 500, and it is probably a good deal lower
than this.

Toxoplasmosis comes from handling cat litter. Pass
this chore over to someone else before you start a pregnancy, or work out some way of doing it so there is
no chance of contact. The parasite is also occasionally
found in the feces of dogs, rabbits, and pet birds. The

woman with primary toxoplasmosis may miscarry or her baby have birth defects of various kinds, including abnormalities of the brain and hydrocephalus. The chances are, however, that even then the baby will be all right, since eight out of ten babies of mothers with this disease have no symptoms at all.

The risks of a woman having German measles in the first three months of pregnancy are well known, and girls are vaccinated against rubella when at school. Women in their thirties may not have had rubella vaccine, and some will not have had the disease or built up immunity to it. Two or three out of every ten babies born to mothers who have German measles in the first three months of pregnancy either die, have a heart defect, or are blind or deaf. This is a chilling statistic and is why termination is offered to any woman who has the infection at the beginning of pregnancy.

Some American studies show that being in a sauna can be dangerous in early pregnancy if your body tem-

RISK OF GERMAN MEASLES AFFECTING THE FETUS[11]

Stage of Pregnancy from Last Period	Risk of Severe Defect
in first 4 weeks	33%
5–8 weeks	25%
9–12 weeks	9%
13–16 weeks	4%
17–30 weeks	1%

perature gets very high and *remains* high.[12] In Scandinavia people having saunas always get into cold water (or roll in the snow) after. For this reason very high temperatures, an extremely hot bath, or lying under a sun lamp for a long time are best avoided. Your own comfort is probably the best guide here. If you run a high fever and think you may be pregnant, it is probably better to take aspirin to get the temperature down, in spite of the disadvantages of aspirin (see page 33), than to allow the fever to continue unabated. If the fever is not high enough to demand anything other than plenty of fluids, a cool room, and perhaps a bag of ice cubes at the back of your neck or at your temples, it may be best to avoid aspirin and other fever-reducing drugs. You are the best person to decide.

Your Life-Style

It is sometimes thought that this kind of information should not be available to women because it makes them unnecessarily anxious. My own view is that I value the facts, that it is my body and my baby, and if I am to understand treatment or investigations proposed, I need information if I am to act as an adult rather than a child.

Moreover, having this kind of information must affect decisions about my life-style, things I do every day, which have nothing to do with medical treatment and of which the obstetrician may be unaware. Part of preparing for a baby is to think through the way I live so that I can provide the best start possible for that new human being.

Women often wonder about exercise...

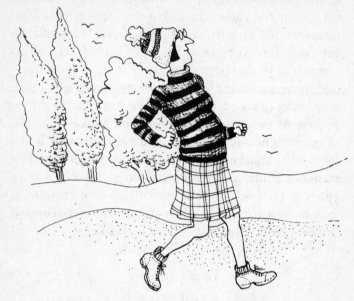

long walks...

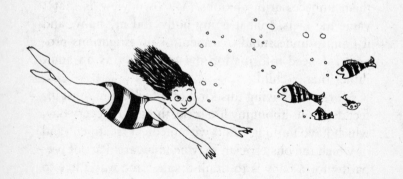

...swimming

Planning Ahead for Pregnancy

Women often wonder about exercise and whether they should slow down on or give up swimming, hill climbing, long walks, and cycle rides, or other athletic activities. Research suggests that if you are physically fit you will have developed physiological mechanisms which allow a fetus to tolerate circulatory and respiratory changes occurring with strenuous exercise. Your own feelings are probably the best guide in this.[13] The changes that usually occur to cope with exercise during pregnancy are like those during regular athletic training; there is increased cardiac output, stroke volume, heart rate, and blood volume. When you are really exerting yourself placental blood flow decreases, but the baby takes more oxygen from your blood. Once you have finished exercising more blood flows through the placenta to the baby than before.

Eating for Two

If you think what an Eskimo mother eats and compare this with a Masai mother's diet, both of whom bear healthy babies, you realize that no strict rules can be laid down about what you should eat and that neither the Eskimo woman's whale blubber nor the Masai blood mixed with milk are essential items of nutrition! Most women benefit, however, from two helpings of a protein food each day. Be generous with fluids, too, since this keeps your bladder and kidneys working well. There is no need to drink milk, though if it is only a matter of disliking it there are many ways of disguising it in other dishes. It used to be thought that liver was a near-perfect food for expectant mothers, in order to prevent anemia and give protein. But the liver and kidneys are like filters in an animal's body, and some modern methods of stock-rearing and of fattening up animals with hormone-laced feed for quick sale introduce doubts on this score. Eat whole-grain bread and brown rice rather than white.

A salad as a main course each day is a good rule, with a side salad at another meal. Vegetables make a good main dish with the addition of cheese, eggs, or both, or have a thick vegetable soup followed by whole-wheat or rye bread with cheese. Potatoes are an excellent source of vitamin C if cooked in their skins. A baked potato stuffed with soft cheese with herbs together with a coleslaw of finely chopped Dutch cabbage with apples and nuts makes a good meal. Have some uncooked fruit every day. Oranges, tangerines, tomatoes, strawberries, and cantaloupe are all rich in vitamin C, and since this vitamin is not stored in the body, it has to be taken regularly.

Avoid junk foods, including carbonated drinks, packaged mixes, bottled sauces, candy bars, and ready-prepared desserts (just look at the list of ingredients to see why) and so-called ice cream. Cut out sugar added to drinks and keep sugar consumption down. It is not a bad idea to go though the cupboards in the kitchen and throw out refined foods such as white flour and the containers you collect at the back of the shelf half full of things you never liked anyway. Bear in mind, though, that you probably have a partner who likes his food, too, and a drastic change may be met with resistance. A new cookbook which specializes in recipes for whole foods, but without being self-consciously "improving," may inspire both of you to experiment with dishes.

If a man has not enjoyed cooking before, now is the time to begin. He needs to be able to produce nutritious and attractive meals quickly, without fuss, and to clear up afterwards. I have sometimes seen it suggested that after a baby is born women should be content to feed their families on things out of cans, hamburgers and french fries, frozen dinners, and Chinese takeouts. Yet nutrition during breastfeeding is very important if a woman is to feel fit and others in the family are to enjoy their meals.

It often starts long before that stage, too, if she has early-morning sickness and evening nausea in the first months of pregnancy. Starvation makes this worse. One way of coping with it is to have frequent nibbles of nutritious foods. So maybe planning for a pregnancy should include a man's attendance at a course of cooking classes!

3

—◆—

Will the Baby
Be All Right?

There are two procedures the older woman having a baby is likely to be offered. One is ultrasound, in which very-high-frequency sound waves, with frequencies too high to be detected by our ears, are bounced off a solid object (in this case the baby) and show up as dots tracing the shape of the baby on a screen. The woman may be asked to attend the test with a full bladder so that the uterus is pushed upward. She lies down, her abdomen is oiled, and a metal arm is moved over her uterus. The whole thing takes about ten minutes.

The other investigation is amniocentesis. After a pain-killing injection given in the lower part of the abdomen, a sample of the amniotic fluid in which the baby floats in pregnancy is drawn off through a needle inserted through the mother's abdominal wall and into the uterus. This fluid contains cast-off cells from the fetus, which can then be grown to form a culture.

Will the Baby Be All Right?

Amniocentesis is a method of ruling out about forty different possible abnormalities in the baby, including spina bifida, when part of the spinal column is exposed, and Down's syndrome, or mongolism. It is used in association with the ultrasound scan. Scans are employed routinely in many hospitals now. Sound waves can confirm pregnancy from about six weeks. Besides ruling out abnormalities such as a tubal pregnancy, they show the fetal heart beating and fetal movements; whether you are having more than one baby; and, if employed in a series, can be used to assess the baby's growth and the relation of the baby to the mother's pelvis. They tend to be used increasingly to take the place of information which the mother already has and which she is perfectly capable of telling the doctor. In fact, in some hospitals there seems to be a basic distrust of everything the patient says, and reliance is put entirely on machines. Their wholesale use for apparently trivial reasons ("You can have a couple of scans," one obstetrician said, "they're a lot of fun") might be questioned if only because they diminish women's sense of competence about what is happening to them and imply that the mother is a passive object of care.

Though ultrasound is probably a great deal safer than X rays, it must be remembered that these were used for many years in obstetrics without anyone questioning their safety, and it was only after they were being employed routinely in some consultant units to measure pelvic capacity that they were found to be carcinogenic. Tests done on ultrasound suggest that there is no hidden danger, but time may teach us differently. We can be fairly positive but never altogether sure.

It is important to state this in spite of the fact that women often like having scans and insist on them. They make the pregnancy more real, and some, unsure whether or not they want the baby, start the process of bonding with the unborn child on seeing its outlines on the screen. "It was fascinating to see the tiny arms and legs pounding away vigorously even before I could feel any movements," said one woman. "I couldn't have faced an abortion after that; it would have been a terrible decision!"

Calculating the Risks

Though an older mother is at a slightly increased risk of having a baby with a congenital malformation, there is no specific reason why she should be more likely to bear a child with malformation of the central nervous system, such as spina bifida. There is an increased risk of having a Down's syndrome baby as one gets older, however, and the chances can be calculated statistically.

Women having late pregnancies are often very frightened of the possibility of having a mentally handicapped baby and particularly that they might bear one that survives for many years. "I don't know how we'd cope . . . it's the worst and most worrying question of all. Will our life become 'lifeless' for ten, twenty years . . . will we 'not exist' because the child doesn't really mentally exist?" Sometimes pregnant women dread this thought so much that they cannot talk about it, as if, somehow, the words could create the fact. They may dream about having a baby which is not "right," though the mental pictures with which they disguise the image of the baby mean that they may not see the dream as anything related to the pregnancy. Dreams about having done shoddy work or produced an object which is imperfect and which is criticized by others (often people in authority or in uniform) seem to be one way in which a woman wraps up her fears of having an abnormal baby. These dreams, when remembered, produce a wave of distress which seems out of all proportion to the incidents which occurred. Sometimes the dream is about baby animals which are disposed of or drowned because other people decide they are not good enough or unwanted. Dreams of losing a part of one's own body which has something wrong with it can also be dreams about the baby. It may be a tooth, limb, or anything else. In pregnancy, especially after you feel the first movements, the baby is like a part of yourself, and birth itself may seem like mutilation.

Though it cannot be inferred that all women are anxious about bearing a handicapped baby, knowing that disturbing and often very vivid dreams are a normal part of pregnancy and that you share the experience with many other women can be reassuring, if only because you then feel less odd. Women often do not talk about these things together, because they are afraid they will be upset and even introduce ideas into other pregnant women's minds and start them worrying. In fact, a substratum of anxiety, a sense of "What if . . . ? How could I cope if . . . ?" is common in pregnancy and can be a useful mental preparation for the psychological challenges which come with being a mother. None of your anxiety is being wasted. It is all grist to the mill.

Women who are feeling fit during pregnancy may be less nagged by doubt about the baby being normal because they feel their bodies are working well. Some are vibrant with health and well-being and better than they ever have been before. Many older mothers are surprised by this and describe with delight long walks in the country, swimming until late pregnancy, enjoying sex (sometimes in a new way), and having softer skin and shinier hair than usual.

It can be very different for a woman who spends much of the first three months of pregnancy with continual nausea and vomiting or feeling exhausted and worn out. She asks herself whether this must not be harming the baby and is it a sign that something is wrong with it. Her anxiety is increased until it may become part of a spiral which is not only the result of her digestive disturbance and tiredness, but in turn tends to increase it. When a rundown state persists after twelve weeks or so and is not cured by extra rest and sleep, it often continues until about the sixteenth week, the time when amniocentesis is performed, and disappears after. Once the woman knows that her baby is not suffering from Down's syndrome she can begin to relax and enjoy her pregnancy.

It is also different with women who have lost a previous baby. One whose last baby had lived for only a week and who is seven months pregnant says, "I have either had, or imagined I had, every possible complication there is. . . . My husband and I have only just started discussing possible names and where on earth there is going to be room for a crib in our bulging house. I cannot take that final step of going shopping for the baby. A few weeks before, a friend said to me, 'So you've finally accepted that you're pregnant,' and I realized that no one apart from the children had really been allowed to talk about it."

Keeping the Secret

Many women do not feel they can tell other people, work colleagues and members of the family, about the coming baby until after amniocentesis. It is almost as if they are not having a baby at all, in spite of all the physical changes. To have to cope with morning sickness, or evening sickness (which is almost as common), not be able to go more than a couple of hours without a cookie or a banana, feel unutterably weary and drag through each day longing for bed, and then not be able to sleep without interruption at night because of pressure on one's bladder and needing to go to the bathroom, all while the pregnancy is hidden from friends and relatives, can be an intolerable burden.

Accidental conception itself may make the older expectant mother feel that something must be wrong with the baby. It is as if *thinking* about starting a baby made it safer. This holds good if it means giving up smoking and having sensible nutrition before conceiving. But it does not mean that the happy accident puts a baby at risk. Phyllis felt that her baby's conception had been "freakish." She had been working very hard, switching between two demanding jobs, and her husband was just over the flu. Amniocentesis set her fears to rest. Even the woman who already has a family may have fears that this time it is not going to work out as it should: "When you have two or three healthy children, you wonder if you are pushing your luck to have another."

When at last it is known that the chances of the baby being mentally handicapped are very slight indeed and the pregnancy can be given social recognition, the whole thing becomes easier. Many women say they felt a load off their minds. One woman who had not recognized that she was at all anxious said, "I felt as if a great weight had been lifted and I realized just how worried I had been." No tests can assure you that the baby is perfect, however, though they can rule out specific abnormalities. Amniocentesis can detect chromosomal abnormalities, neural tube defects such as anencephaly and spina bifida, and many errors of metabolism. Screening for central nervous system defects is done prior to amniocentesis, however, and you only go on to have amniocentesis for further investigation if the alpha-fetoprotein level is high in a sample of your blood.

Alpha-fetoprotein (AFP) is a substance rather like the albumin appearing in the urine of the woman who is developing preeclampsia, which is synthesized by the baby's liver. It passes into the amniotic fluid and from there into the mother's blood. Levels double every five weeks during the middle trimester of pregnancy. There is no level which clearly defines an abnormal pregnancy and AFP concentration varies with pregnancy, going steadily up until it reaches its maximum level at about thirty weeks. Between the sixteenth and eighteenth weeks the gap between normal and high levels of AFP is greatest, so this is the best time to measure it. The dating of your pregnancy is important, because a high level might mean that you were later in pregnancy than you thought. It is also high if you are carrying more than one baby. AFP testing is done routinely in some areas and you may not know you have had it. It is worth asking.

With Down's syndrome, however, AFP testing is not enough, and the only way at present to find out if your baby has it is to have an amniocentesis. There is no point in having this done if you would not want the pregnancy terminated anyway, so it is important to think through how you feel about this in advance. Whatever decision you make, it is *your* choice, not the doctor's.

Down's Syndrome

Ninety-five percent of cases of Down's syndrome are age-related and result from a chromosomal disorder called a "trisomy," when there is an extra, unpaired chromosome. It is estimated that about half of all babies with Down's syndrome are miscarried early in pregnancy. Though the overall incidence of having a baby with Down's syndrome is one in 650 live births, in fact chances are low while you are still in your twenties and only start creeping up after thirty-five.

Mother's age	Approximate risk[1] of affected child 1 per 1000 live births
20	1 in 2000
25	1 in 1205
30	1 in 885
35	1 in 365
36	1 in 290
37	1 in 225
38	1 in 180
39	1 in 140
40	1 in 109
41	1 in 85
42	1 in 70
43	1 in 50
44	1 in 40
45	1 in 32
46	1 in 25
47	1 in 20
48	1 in 15
49	1 in 12

There are other chromosome abnormalities, however, which are also age-related, and when these are looked at too, the chances of an affected fetus are higher.

There is a strong case for having amniocentesis if you are forty or older. Before that time the best action is not always clear, since the investigation itself introduces a risk to the pregnancy, and between one and two babies in each 100 are miscarried as a result of the test. Rarely, very rarely, the lumbar puncture needle used to extract the fluid through the mother's abdom-

ALL CHROMOSOME ABNORMALITIES[2]

Mother's age	Incidence
25	1 in 527
30	1 in 476
35	1 in 204
40	1 in 73
45	1 in 23

inal and uterine walls punctures the baby, causing injury. This should never happen when an ultrasound scan is done immediately before and the position of the fetus accurately located during the test. Even so, women are often anxious that the baby may be damaged. Rosalyn said she could not face the idea of amniocentesis because, though she wanted to know whether or not the baby had Down's syndrome, she would go through the rest of her pregnancy worrying that the needle had slipped into its eye, and she had tried so hard to get pregnant for so long that she didn't want to take any risks; all she wanted was a baby, whether or not it had Down's syndrome. Since she felt this, it was obviously the right choice for her to refuse amniocentesis, though she was forty-one.

The older woman is more likely to have fibroids in her uterus, and the obstetrician may advise one who is between thirty-five and forty against having an amniocentesis in the presence of a fibroid in case she miscarries. If you have had previous miscarriages it is possible that this might also make the amniocentesis that much trickier, though there is no way of being sure.

Unfortunately the test cannot be done until sixteen weeks, about fourteen weeks from the probable date of conception. The two extra weeks are added to date you back to the first day of your last menstrual period, which is the only date doctors think you are likely to remember accurately. Some women make up this date for convenience. If you really are very unsure it is best to be honest about it, since it can affect the results of the test. Before that time there is not enough fluid. Leaving it for more than two weeks later would entail a more difficult abortion should you decide on termination, since the chromosome culture and analysis takes another two to three weeks.

Testing the Waters

It is important to realize before amniocentesis that it is not a question of popping in a needle like a coin in a slot and coming up with an answer. You will probably feel anxious, and it is not a bad idea to go with a friend, especially if you know someone who has been through it before. Liz, for example, went with a friend who was two months ahead of her, "and we were able to boost each other afterward"; all went well, but she says she found it worrying when the woman before her came out saying that they could not get enough fluid after trying four times and she had to return in two weeks.

"I disliked intensely the sensation of the needle going

in to retrieve some fluid. The doctor made two attempts to get some fluid and still couldn't get any," Angela said. "I would have had to go back two weeks later. I decided against it. The incident made me feel tremendously protective toward my child. The needle in my stomach felt so threatening."

Another woman expressed her distaste of amniocentesis as a reaction to an intrusion on the intimacy of her pregnancy:

"I felt the baby's privacy had been invaded with this needle going in to its amniotic sac."

Helen says that amniocentesis was "an appalling experience," made worse because she dreaded it and knows she "tensed up." It wasn't helped by the lecture from the doctor on the risks of amniocentesis and being asked to sign the consent form, though this should always be done.

Ultrasound is used to locate the pool of amniotic fluid and the position of the placenta first. Your abdomen is covered with sterile cloths except where first the injection for the local anesthetic and then the amniocentesis needle is to be introduced. There is a prick which you cannot feel and the fluid is drawn off. Occasionally it has to be done again but cannot be done immediately because the uterus has started to contract. But if you lie quietly for fifteen minutes or so, these contractions will fade away. Do not conclude that you have started labor.

Many women find it all far simpler than they expected. Emma said that her consultant introduced the needle very low down, after shaving off a small patch of pubic hair.

I felt a couple of tiny pinpricks and thought they were just the preliminaries. The consultant commented to the midwife that the abdomen was rather tough and he was having difficulty getting the needle through. I still thought this was for the local anesthetic. Then I felt a fluttering sensation deep inside. It suddenly dawned on me that this was the actual amniocentesis procedure itself.

You may find that the needle leaves a painful bruise, especially if another insertion had to be made, since air may then be introduced. It will have disappeared after a few days and does not mean that any harm has come to the baby, though it may be uncomfortable if you have an older child climbing all over you.

The baby's heart will be checked before you have the amniocentesis and again afterward, and it is a comfort if you have a chance to see the baby moving on the ultrasound scan after the amniocentesis has been performed. You can ask for this if it is not suggested.

If the mother is Rh-negative, since there is a chance of some of the baby's blood crossing the placenta, she is given an injection to prevent the build-up of antibodies in her blood which may adversely affect the baby. After amniocentesis, take it easy if you can for the next twelve hours.

The Results

There follows the stressful period of waiting two weeks or more before you get the diagnosis. Anna said this was "horrible," and she delayed applying for a course on having a baby until she got the results. She felt in limbo. One woman, who had to wait a full month, commented that it was "horrid, like waiting for exam results." In about five percent of cases a culture cannot be grown, and the test either has to be done again or, if as sometimes happens, the woman is more than twenty weeks pregnant, it may be decided to skip it and she still does not know one way or the other.

Some women stress that articles in magazines and TV programs give the impression that amniocentesis and ultrasound scans are processes in which the woman participates, has a chance to ask questions, and can learn something about her baby. They found that they were expected to lie down, be quiet, and do what they were told. "My questions were either ignored or dismissed," one said. Another, "very excited at the prospect of seeing the fetus," said that the radiographer gossiped to her assistant all the way through. "The only consolation I could draw was that she was looking at the screen and there were no sharp intakes of breath! . . . I had the feeling that a tremendous opportunity for letting the mother in on what was happening was missed." She did manage to see the scan herself, but "for all I know I could have been looking at a shoulder of lamb!"

Jan said she felt "very scared" at having a scan, and when she found she was alone with two technicians she had never seen before, was worried that they would not know what to tell her if something was wrong: "I didn't want to see the fetus, was very tense, and felt my relationship with the baby was private." She is one of many women who wished they had taken their husbands with them.

Ultrasound is used to narrow down the chances of a baby with a neural tube defect being missed, or one who is normal being aborted when AFP levels are high, since open lesions can usually be detected on the screen.

Fetal cells obtained from amniocentesis will also tell whether you are having a boy or a girl. This is only important medically if there is the possibility of a sex-linked inherited disease, such as hemophilia or Duchenne's muscular dystrophy. It is usually up to you whether or not you wish to be told the sex of your baby. Some women want to keep it a surprise and believe that knowing in advance makes the pregnancy less "normal." Occasionally an obstetrician has a policy of never telling a woman because he or she does not trust the woman not to try and terminate the pregnancy if the baby is the "wrong" sex. With technological power comes new responsibilities, ones which should be exercised by parents and not only by professionals.

A Termination

When a woman has already felt her baby moving within her, coping with the knowledge that it may have Down's syndrome or a central nervous system anomaly can make her feel very alone. Some women say that everything they do comes automatically, and when the news is given them, it is like pressing a button to start an inevitable process for which they were mentally prepared all along. It is not so much a question of "why is this baby abnormal?" but "how could I have ever thought that I could bear a normal baby?" Most have not revealed the pregnancy to people at work and many

56

have not told close family members either, so they feel bound to put a brave face on it and carry on as usual.

Many also say they would appreciate someone who understands to talk with in between receiving the news and having the abortion. Some hospitals provide counselors. Rarely a group of women who have gone through the experience themselves is available to offer one-to-one emotional support.

Suzanne was told by the hospital registrar that at thirty-seven she did not come within the age group for which amniocentesis was available, and he was unwilling to agree to it. "I was strong and experienced," she says, "and asked if I might have an appointment with the consultant, who readily agreed to make the arrangements." She went back three weeks later for the results: "I had deliberately resisted any involvement with the fetus—difficult—but I knew I would terminate if anything was grossly wrong." The consultant told her the baby had Down's syndrome. "Though I had long imagined facing this news and slipped into the pattern I had prepared for myself, I was emotionally affected more than I expected. . . . We coped with paperwork and I asked for a quick admission." There was only twenty-four hours to wait, but she wonders how she would have managed this without a supportive husband and GP. The abortion was efficiently and sympathetically done. She feels that someone should have told her that at this stage of pregnancy her body would react as if she had delivered a live child and that she would lactate.

In the past a woman who had delivered a dead baby would have had estrogen pills to suppress her milk.

This is no longer done because of the risk of postpartum hemorrhage (bleeding after delivery) and thromboembolism (a blood clot which breaks off and blocks a blood vessel). It was never particularly effective anyway, and when the estrogen was stopped the women often became engorged again. A better way is to bind the breasts tightly or wear a good bra, use cold compresses (ice cubes in a face towel or large handkerchief are comforting), and take analgesics if the breasts are painful. Vitamin B6 in 200-milligram doses has been shown to reduce engorgement for nine out of ten women. It is effective in about eleven hours and should be taken for five days.[3]

Expressing milk merely encourages the milk supply, but on the third and fourth days, when the breasts are likely to be most hot and swollen, kneeling in a hot bath with the breasts suspended in the water allows the milk to stream out without providing extra stimulation.

To have milk pouring from your breasts when you have no baby to feed is as if your whole body is weeping. For some women there is a peculiar comfort in being able to surrender their bodies completely to grief in this way. Suzanne decided not to attempt another pregnancy:

Physically I feel able to cope with termination again but it was such a difficult emotional experience I'm not certain I would want it. I had expected to value life a lot less after depriving something of life, but exactly the opposite reaction occurred.

Will the Baby Be All Right?

Other women have gone on, after a breathing space and a time for grieving for the lost baby, to embark on another pregnancy; they have had an amniocentesis again and have given birth to normal, healthy babies with enormous gratitude and delight. They sometimes say that they did not really let the grieving go till they had had another baby. "I didn't get the longing out of my system until Deirdre was born."

Sometimes a loving husband, anxious to protect his wife from the suffering involved, does not agree to another pregnancy. A woman may see this as if he has no confidence in her and is telling her she cannot cope. The result can be that she resents him for treating her like a child and for what she may interpret as an insensitive and cruel rejection. The two move into their separate emotional worlds.

This was what happened to Sally and Tom. She wrote:

> He was adamant that another disaster could not be allowed to occur and within three months had a vasectomy. He was totally unable to comprehend my wish for another baby which might lead to an abortion and more sorrow. We sought advice on artificial insemination but he backed out. So we are now left, often at loggerheads, and at best pushing away the fact that I still resent him.

This kind of pain can be experienced even when there are other living children. The Down's syndrome baby was Sally's twelfth child.

After she had lost the baby one woman realized she had shut herself away from her husband's pain because it was more than she could handle and merely sharpened her own ordeal. She exerted a tremendous effort of will to be cheerful because she wanted to show him and her parents that she had "come to terms" with the experience. Tears welled up when she had locked the bathroom door, but she never allowed herself to cry in front of her husband. Looking back on it, she feels she made things more difficult for both of them. "After about a week I realized he was suffering with no support from me. I'd actually forgotten I wasn't suffering alone." Then they began to cling to each other and to share the grieving. This itself brought healing.

4

Prenatal Care

U nderstanding what goes on during prenatal care is
important if you are to have accurate information
on which to base decisions. At your first appointment,
tests and history-taking will be more time-consuming
than later appointments. You will be interviewed by a
doctor or by his nurse (or in some hospitals by a staff
doctor), and it would be a good idea to contact him

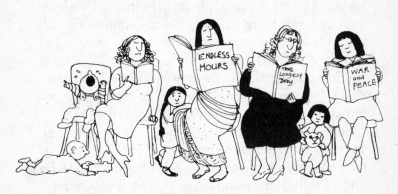

Take a good book or team up with a friend

or her if any worries develop or if you have unanswered questions. The doctor or nurse will ask the first day of your last menstrual period (LMP) and whether you have a regular menstrual cycle and its length. This is so that the expected date of delivery (EDD) can be worked out, by adding seven days and nine months to that day. Avoid guessing a date for the start of your period earlier than it may have been, as induction of labor may be proposed because you appear to be overdue.

She will want to know about operations and illnesses you have had, including urinary infections such as cystitis, German measles (rubella), sexually transmitted diseases such as nonspecific urethritis and yeast infections, and any medicines you are taking. The obstetric history includes all previous births and abortions, whether they were spontaneous (miscarriages) or induced. Let her know if you had any pregnancy problems or birth complications before. You may also be asked questions about the health of your own family and whether any of them suffer from high blood pressure or diabetes, for example, and she may ask whether there are, say, twins or triplets in the family. She will probably ask if you smoke, and if so, how many a day and how many alcoholic drinks you usually have. If you are not married there may be detailed questions about housing and your plans for the future, and you can also ask to have a talk with the social worker.

Someone will weigh you, as they will at subsequent visits, too, and measure your height. The range of possible weight gain in pregnancy is wide, and there is no single "right" or "normal" gain. The largest weekly gains usually occur in mid-pregnancy. If you gain a good deal then, it does not mean that you will continue to put on as much until the end of pregnancy. This is not the time to diet by cutting down on nutrition, though if you are gaining weight too rapidly for comfort, it is a good idea to omit carbohydrate foods and, in particular, sugar, including the sauces, canned foods, drinks, and other dishes in which there is invisible sugar. Though if you gain little weight you are more likely to have a lightweight baby than if you put on a lot, women who gain none at all have babies who are only 9 to 12 ounces less than those who gain a great deal.

The urine specimen is another regular part of the prenatal visit. It is tested for the presence of glucose (which occurs in diabetes and prediabetic conditions), protein (one of the signs of preeclampsia), and bacteria (produced by a urinary infection). You may be asked to produce a midstream sample of urine, which is done by interrupting the stream of urine with a strong pelvic floor contraction and then letting the second flow of urine go into the container provided.

Your blood pressure will also be taken, using a sphygmomanometer. In early pregnancy blood pressure is down to lower than normal: the upper figure, the systolic, a little bit, but the lower, the diastolic, well below the nonpregnant level. During the seventh or eighth month the diastolic pressure rises to your more usual level, and under stress the upper figure, which is readily affected by strong emotion, may be high (if you are anxious or angry or have had to rush to your appointment, for example). If you find out what your blood pressure is at thirty or thirty-two weeks when relaxed, you will have a rough idea of what is normal for you.

Preeclampsia

In mild preeclampsia, which occurs in about ten percent of all pregnancies during the last few weeks, without harming the baby, blood pressure rises to about 140/90. The lower figure is the important one, as it is the resting pressure between heartbeats. In about two percent of pregnancies preeclampsia is severe and the upper figure approaches 160, the lower 100, even when you are resting in a bed. First-time mothers are more likely to develop preeclampsia than those having second or subsequent babies. Even if you have only had a miscarriage before, you are probably protected from preeclampsia, though not if you are pregnant by a new partner.

At the first appointment your heart is usually checked with a stethoscope, and at the same time breasts and nipples are examined. If your nipples are inverted there is a good chance that their shape will change during pregnancy, and even if there is little alteration, once you get the baby firmly fixed onto your breast he or she will draw the nipple into the back of the mouth and mold it into the right shape. If you want to help the whole process, suggest to your partner that love play should include plenty of manual and oral stimulation of your nipples. You do not need to do anything else.

At the first visit some blood is taken so that your

hemoglobin level can be checked (if below ten at the twelfth week of pregnancy you are anemic); your blood group is noted in case you need a transfusion and so that any problems associated with being Rh-negative or ABO can be anticipated. The blood is also tested for venereal disease, antibodies to rubella, and in many cases, after sixteen weeks, for levels of alpha-fetoprotein. You are given an internal examination to feel the state of the uterus and the cervix, and at the same time a cervical Pap smear is taken to detect any precancerous cells (or this may be done at your postnatal checkup).

When you are up on the table to be examined by the doctor or midwife, he or she may look at your legs to see if you have varicose veins and, later in pregnancy, for any swelling (edema, a sign of fluid retention). The abdomen is palpated to see where the top of the womb lies. The height of the fundus (the top of the uterus) in relation to the pubic bone at the front of the pelvis is one way of estimating the length of gestation.

From twenty-eight weeks the doctor or midwife checks how the baby is lying and whether it is presenting by head or buttocks. They will listen to the fetal heartbeat, and if you would like to hear it, too, ask to do so. If you are Rh-negative there will be more blood tests from this time to see if you are developing antibodies.

You may also be asked to give urine over twenty-four hours to test the function of the placenta by measuring the estriol it produces. When estriol levels fall, it is a sign that the placenta is entering its old age. A single specimen can give no idea at all of your estriol levels, since output varies at different times within the twenty-four hours. If for any reason you are on antibiotics or corticosteroids (for severe asthma, for example), the urinary estriol level will fall, and a low level does not mean that placental function is poor. Sometimes these tests are done on blood instead of urine. Sometimes even when results of such tests are normal, induction of labor may be proposed "because of your age." There is no need to consent to any procedure for which you do not have adequate explanation.

The Baby's Movements

Studies of mothers' own perceptions of their baby's movements suggest that these may be more precise than measuring the output of hormones. Any measurable changes in the placental output of estrogen *follow* an obvious reduction in the baby's activity.[1]

Through your awareness of your baby's movements, you get to know about and be in touch with it in a very direct way. In the recent past, with the emphasis on modern obstetric technology, the mother's knowledge of her unborn baby's activity, its cycles of sleep and waking, and the location and nature of its movements, has been largely ignored and considered irrelevant beside the "scientific" evidence concerning placental function from urine and blood tests and the ultrasound scans and other ways of getting windows into the womb, which are now employed in almost every obstetric unit. The mother has a unique opportunity, however, to get to know her baby and to be aware of it throughout the twenty-four hours in a way which is impossible for any outsider. Abigail Lewis, writing of her own pregnancy, says of the fetus:

It stretches and turns; its movements gain in power and
direction. Whatever may be your own doubts about
where mankind is heading and what maturity is, the
fetus seems to feel no doubt at all as to what it wants;
and in all that curious, segregated, seemingly static
chunk of a year, you become aware of a new kind of
time, the fetus's time, the slow pushing time of growth.[2]

The fetus is a water-baby in a fluid-filled capsule.
Though the mother does not usually feel movements
till about four and a half months, it is moving before
then. Until the uterus has lifted out of the pelvic cavity
into the abdomen these movements are not felt because
the wall of the uterus has no touch reception. It is only
when it is lying against the abdomen that touch can be
experienced. With very little gravitational pull from the
earth, the fetus in the uterus is like a swimmer under
water, or perhaps more like an astronaut in space.
Movement is easy, and it twists and turns, flips from
side to side, and while there is still room, before the
eighth month of pregnancy, may somersault. It holds
on to its umbilical cord, sometimes sucks its thumb,
sometimes loses the thumb and darts its head from side
to side searching for it again, bounces its head against
the springy pelvic floor muscles when it has dropped
deep into the pelvis, presses its feet against the thick
muscle forming the top of the uterus in a stepping
movement, rubs its eyes with tiny fists, and sometimes
its whole body jerks with hiccups.

Some of these movements may occur in response to
sound. The fetus hears from about the twenty-fifth week
and may react strongly to loud noises and music, es-

pecially to the clash of cymbals or a brass band. At any time from about six weeks before term (the date the baby is expected) the fetus may drop lower into the pelvis and "engage." If it is a snug fit it is then difficult for the fetus to make any big, whole body movements, though it still kicks vigorously. The nature of the movements changes when this happens, unless the fetus is small and the mother's pelvis large, in which case it may stay equally active. The fetus who is lying with its back against its mother's spine may also feel very active, as the limbs are at the front.

It is important to be aware that there may be a qualitative difference in activity when the fetus engages in a vertex (head down) position, facing the mother's side or back, however. If you do not know that this can happen, there may be panic when the movements are more restricted. Some women notice that their babies seem to sleep for longer periods then, too, rather as if the fetus is settled comfortably, like the dormouse in the teapot in *Alice in Wonderland*, and does not want to be disturbed. Perhaps it is a good time for conserving energy ready for labor.

"About a week before the expected date of arrival I thought William had died because he wasn't moving," Antonia says. "I became absolutely hysterical. I walked down a busy downtown street weeping. It took me three tries to get the nurse at the hospital to understand what I was saying, all my emotions were all over the place." She is a single mother and she felt submerged with loneliness: "I really needed someone to lean on then. Wow! Horrific! But the hospital said come up at once, and they put a monitor on the heart and he was just sleeping."

Because women can get so alarmed about not feeling movements, some doctors think it is disturbing for them to be asked to note them. Some obstetricians feel strongly that it is vital to reassure women at all costs and leave the worrying to the professionals. Doctors who believe this tend to favor blood and urine tests which are done and analyzed at the hospital over against anything which a woman can do herself.

Yet no one would suggest that a mother should leave observation of her baby solely to pediatricians once it is born. She is the one in day-to-day contact with her child and, as such, can have more intimate knowledge than anyone who sees the child only for a clinical examination. Even when she does see a professional for advice, common sense tells us that the doctor ought to spend some time finding out what the mother knows about the child and listening to her. It is purely arbitrary to say that a mother should do this *after* birth, but that before the baby has emerged she need not bother herself with the matter and should "leave it to the doctor." While the baby is still inside her, in fact, there is closer contact between the two than they are ever going to experience after delivery.

A Kick Chart

One good way of checking that your baby is doing well in the uterus is to keep a kick chart. It is simple to do, noninvasive, and costs nothing, and can be very useful as you get to the last weeks of your pregnancy, especially if induction is proposed, since you can probably produce evidence that your baby is vigorous. A baby who is moving well when it is awake (and remember that every baby has sleeping times) is *not at risk*. It is best to pick a regular time each day when you know from experience that your baby tends to be active. Most women find that this happens in the evening, when they have a chance to sit down and probably notice movements more readily than when busy and moving about. Antonia, remember, did not feel her baby move once while she was walking up and down the busy downtown street. If she had gone home and got into a bath or put her feet up on the bed she would have probably felt movements in the next hour or so.

Use graph paper, each square representing a half-hour period during your observation time. Shade in the square at which you feel the tenth movement each day. It should occur at approximately the same time each evening, give or take thirty minutes or so.

The result will be a chart that may look something like this:

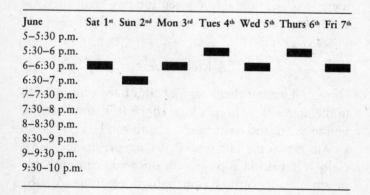

June	Sat 1st	Sun 2nd	Mon 3rd	Tues 4th	Wed 5th	Thurs 6th	Fri 7th
5–5:30 p.m.							
5:30–6 p.m.				■		■	
6–6:30 p.m.	■		■		■		■
6:30–7 p.m.		■					
7–7:30 p.m.							
7:30–8 p.m.							
8–8:30 p.m.							
8:30–9 p.m.							
9–9:30 p.m.							
9:30–10 p.m.							

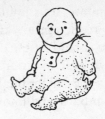

That baby is doing well!

When you are about to start labor, fetal movements may be reduced, and your chart may look like this:

June	Sat 8th	Sun 9th	Mon 10th	Tues 11th
5–5:30 p.m.				
5:30–6 p.m.				
6–6:30 p.m.	�			
6:30–7 p.m.		▬		
7–7:30 p.m.			▬	
7:30–8 p.m.				▬

If at any time you have felt no fetal movement for a full twelve hours, call your obstetrician or the nurse. There is no need to be alarmed, since the baby usually starts kicking soon after, but it is best to take action. One study[3] of sixty-seven women who had no fetal movements for at least twelve hours found that fifty-five of them had healthy babies after a labor which started normally. The other twelve babies were passing meconium (the first contents of the bowel) or had abnormal heart rates, so labor was induced and all were born alive, ten in excellent condition and two with low Apgar ratings at five minutes (the Apgar score is a system of estimating the baby's condition at birth with reference to the heart rate, breathing, muscle tone, color,

71

and response to stimulation). If you notice a fifty percent reduction in kicks continuing over several days you should let the doctor know about it. You are your own best monitor of this, not because you are watching for danger but because you are in touch with your own baby and know your baby better than anyone else.

If the fetus is not moving the doctor will probably decide to do a "nonstress test." Ultrasound stimulates the fetus to move and the heart to speed up, so it is

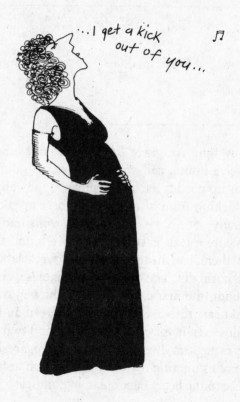

used to record the reactions of the baby. If there is no response it is concluded that the baby is short of oxygen. If the baby starts kicking it is a sign that all is well. If you know that your baby usually reacts to special kinds of music you can try the effects of this even before you go to the hospital. One woman, a singer, said her baby always started moving when she was at a rehearsal or concert, so she could always check how her baby was by bursting into song! If you go past your due date your observation of the baby's kicking is even more important, as careful recording could make all the difference between labor being induced and being able to start naturally.

Every time you are seen in a prenatal appointment, the results are recorded in your medical chart by the nurse and the doctor or midwife. Results of the medical exam, including any lab work, subjects discussed, suggestions made, medications prescribed, etc., are recorded, too. You have the right to see your records if you wish. Although doctors sometimes think this may cause a patient unnecessary anxiety, since the information in the records is all about her body and her baby, it seems reasonable for a pregnant woman to have access to them.

On the next two pages there are some of the abbreviations you may find in them. Some appear with a question mark beside them. You will see that some abbreviations are similar to others. NAD is a very usual entry, yet is like NTD—neural tube defect. If in any doubt about the writing get up the courage to ask the person who wrote it.

THE CLINIC

AF	amniotic fluid
AFP	alpha-fetoprotein (see p. 48)
APH	antepartum hemorrhage
BP	blood pressure
BPD	biparietal diameter, head measurement. This is assessed by ultrasound, the usual method of recording fetal growth. It is most accurate before twenty-four weeks, widely inaccurate after thirty-four weeks. BPD grows 3.4 mm a week at seventeen weeks, slows down to about a third of that at the end of pregnancy.
AROM	artificial rupture of membranes
CPD	cephalopelvic disproportion. The baby will not go through the mother's pelvis.
DPB	diastolic blood pressure (see p. 63)
E1, 2, or 3	estrogen output
EDD/EDC	estimated date of delivery/confinement
FBS	fetal blood sample
Fe	iron
FH/FHH	fetal heart heard
FHR	fetal heart rate
GA	general anesthetic
GTT	glucose tolerance test, done if there is suspected diabetes
Hb	hemoglobin (see p. 65)
H/T	hypertension, high blood pressure
HVS	high vaginal swab
IUCD	intrauterine contraceptive device, loop or coil
IUD	intrauterine death
IUGR	intrauterine growth retardation
IUT	intrauterine transfusion, very rare
IV	intravenous
LMP	last menstrual period
CS	cesarean section
L/S	lecithin-sphingomyelin ratio, used to test maturity of fetal lungs, e.g., when mother has diabetes

MSU	midstream specimen of urine
NAD	nothing abnormal detected
NTD	neural tube defect
OA	occiput anterior, baby lying head down, facing mother's back. Most favorable position.
LOA	left occiput anterior
ROA	right occiput anterior
OCT	oxytocin challenge test. Intravenous infusion of oxytocin while monitoring fetal heart to see how baby responds to strong contractions.
OP	occiput posterior. Baby lying head down, facing mother's front. Expect long first stage of labor, with backache. Keep upright and moving, if possible.
LOP	left occiput posterior
ROP	right occiput posterior
OT	occiput transverse. Baby lying head down, the side of its head toward mother's front. May move to anterior or posterior.
PE$_2$/PGE$_2$	prostaglandin used in induction
PET	preeclamptic toxemia (see p. 64)
PPH	postpartum hemorrhage
RE	rectal examination
POP	persistent occiput posterior
SBP	systolic blood pressure (see p. 63)
SVD	spontaneous vaginal delivery/spontaneous vertex delivery
T$_3$R	test of thyroid function
VE	vaginal examination

5

Doctors

One great advantage in being older and more experienced in coping with people can be that a woman is more skilled and confident in finding out what she needs to know about the medical system, maneuvering her way through it and getting what she wants. This may have to start when the pregnancy is first confirmed. One woman, very happy to be pregnant by a man with whom she had lived for two years, went to a gynecologist to make sure that all was well. He told her she was definitely pregnant and then said, "When do you want the abortion?" "Abortion?" she said. "I want this baby." "Oh," he replied, "forty and unmarried. Most unusual." She found she had to convince the doctor that she wanted to go ahead with the pregnancy, an experience that might have thrown a younger woman.

The woman in her thirties or forties is more likely to know where to go to get accurate information, how to sift the evidence, and how to negotiate the kind of childbirth she would like to have, in the setting of her choice. Julie was having her fourth baby at forty. The others had all been born at home, and she wanted this one at home, too. "I merely told them that unless there were pressing medical contraindications, I should stay at home. One said that they might not have a midwife available. I said that didn't deter me." He said no more and a midwife duly appeared. "I did need to have a certain amount of stubbornness," she added. Another woman had fully intended to have her baby in the hospital, but one week before the due date visited the delivery suite and decided then and there that she was not prepared to have her baby in such surroundings and had a home birth after all.

After a four-hour wait at a prenatal clinic, Caroline, who wanted a natural birth, was told by a consultant that she was to be induced, that she would need an epidural anesthetic because induced labor was always more painful, that she must make up her mind about this immediately, and that a first labor was always at least twenty-four hours. At first she could not cope with this situation, but when she arrived home weeping and distressed, her husband took immediate action, phoned the consultant, and explained that she wanted no drugs unless essential. The induction went well and no painkillers were necessary, though she asked for an epidural just as she was entering transition, but on learning that she was almost fully dilated decided it was not necessary. "The anesthetist came back to give me 'just a little jab to help the pain.' John asked what was in this 'jab,' and the anesthetist said, 'Demerol.' We said, 'No thank you.' " The baby slipped out shortly after, and Caroline was delighted to have a natural birth without drugs. Her husband had been her ally and support in this, and together they had done it. Summing up, she says, "The process of labor and giving birth was highly satisfactory, partly I'm sure due to the fact that my husband and I asserted our rights and developed a very positive relationship with the midwife."

In fact, for most women it is not as straightforward as that. Many say they find prenatal clinics appalling and communication inadequate, and the assumptions that doctors make about their passive role as patients lead them to feel frustrated and helpless. Carole lives in an industrial town and had shared care between midwives and doctors. She contrasts the midwives' clinic, where it is easy to discuss worries and ask questions, with the physicians' clinic, where women sit for long periods and "never see the same person twice." In fact, she says she once sat there for two and a half hours. "The doctor puts in an appearance, says, 'Good afternoon, is everything all right . . . I'll just listen to your tummy . . . thank you, see you next week.' " She never managed to extract any information about her pregnancy from the obstetrician, but nevertheless continued to attend the clinic to undergo this ritual.

Another woman, who might be considered competent in communication since she is a postdoctoral developmental psychologist engaged in research, says that she had to "squeeze every single piece of information" out of the doctor and was "appalled at the whole business." Joanne refused to go to the hospital clinic after being "treated like a moron" and had appointments with her physician instead. Dorothy, having her third baby at forty, insisted on a home birth after her experience of the prenatal clinic:

> I was handed a booklet urging me to bring any worries to the doctor. When I am ushered in to him he addresses his questions to me with his back turned while filling in my form. He turns only to look at my bulge and my vulva and never addresses any remarks to my face at all. At what point does one break in with one's inmost anxieties? Perhaps I should have gone in a frog mask just to see if he would notice?

Feeling Old

Being surrounded by much younger women in the clinic can also make you feel older than you are. One woman, very conscious of her gray hairs, was told by the nurse to "run along home, dear, we haven't time for grand-mas today." (A letter of apology arrived afterward.) On the other hand, many women are pleasantly surprised to find that they are not alone in being older mothers and that what one woman called "obstetric geriatrics" are becoming commonplace. Clinic staff, however, may, often inadvertently, suggest that pregnancy and labor are going to be especially difficult. One expectant mother of thirty-seven said that throughout her pregnancy she felt that the famous teaching hospital she attended treated her as "a freak."

Nancy, aged thirty-six, said that she was trying to find out at the hospital whether she could arrange a Leboyer-style delivery and have an early discharge. They told her to speak to the head nurse to find out about hospital policy. The appointment for which she asked was long delayed, so she asked the obstetrician during her next prenatal visit. He said, "Oh, I shouldn't worry about all that if I were you. At your age you are more than likely to spend the last few weeks in the hospital and then to be induced or have a cesarean."

The woman who is having a late baby after a long gap is able to compare the present experience with previous births. If her first children are already in their teens, she spans the time during which there has been a complete medicalization of childbirth. One woman, for example, commented on the contrast between the personal care she was given when she was twenty and felt "rather clever" at having a baby and the impersonal, factory-farm baby production she experienced when she had another baby at forty-two, and remarked how "grim" it is nowadays. Another said: "Pregnancy and childbirth seem to be a nightmare now. People are very afraid and forever worrying about their due date and whether the baby is growing." Several women had such bad experiences with big hospitals when they started second families in their late thirties that they insisted on having subsequent babies in a small hospital or at home and were very glad they did. Some who were in their early thirties had first babies at home. They often found they had to battle for this, though occasionally it was welcomed by the physician. Jill, aged thirty-three, said she went to the doctor "armed with statistics and arguments about the desirability of a home birth . . . whereupon he took all the wind out of my sails by saying, 'Oh, yes, that'll be rather nice. I haven't done one of those for a long time.' " The hospital doctors were a different matter. One made it clear to Jill that "the decision about where to have my baby had nothing to do with me and would be made on my behalf by her. I soon disabused her of that notion and amended the relevant parts she marked on my chart." It is not just that hospital care is sometimes stark and unfriendly; many women feel that the failure to achieve any continuity actually results in second-class or dangerous medicine and obstetrics.

The pregnant woman has a responsibility, for herself and her baby, to discover the choices open to her, weigh their relative advantages, and make sure that everyone knows what she wants. It means that she also has to be sufficiently courageous to complain when necessary and to withdraw her consent for procedures which she is not happy about, unless more convincing arguments are produced. This entails behavior very different from that traditionally considered appropriate to the feminine role, and many women feel acutely uncomfortable with it. They want to please; it feels good to make the doctor smile; they do not want to fuss, or, indeed, to be noticed as different in any way. It is much easier to conform to the doctor's expectations of the "good patient." Diana Scully, in her study of the training of obstetricians and gynecologists in the United States,[1] asked doctors how they would describe a good patient. Their answers emphasized passivity, obedience, and middle-class status. One said: "The main thing is that the patient understands what I say, listens to what I say, does what I say, believes what I say."

Birth Over Thirty

The "Vocal Minority"

The woman who has had the opportunity of education and a career has special responsibilities in this because she is speaking for other women who have not had her advantages and who may be even more at a loss, and more confused and anxious than she is. Yet she has to be prepared for possible hostility or suspicion on the part of the doctor simply *because* she is a middle-class woman asking questions (the medical press tends to call such women the "vocal minority"). The doctor has often been trained to see pregnant women (and most obstetricians are men) only as patients who receive his instructions. He may see the skill of communication as in giving these instructions clearly, rather than as a two-way conversation. And if the patient does not comply, she is "a defaulter."

Ann Oakley, in her book *Subject Women*, writes:

> The idea that it is *women* who cause the deaths of babies—by not going [for prenatal care] (or not going early enough), by smoking, eating the wrong food, having sexual intercourse, not being married, or reading *The Sunday Times*—implicitly acknowledges women's disobedience in doing what *they* think is best for themselves and their babies.[2]

In a footnote she adds that articles published by Oliver and Louise Gillie in *The Sunday Times* of London were often referred to by doctors, in consultations she was observing in a hospital, with women who queried their treatment, as improper sources of information. In fact, any woman who questions treatment on the basis of something she has read may be dismissed with "you mustn't believe everything you read," or castigated with the shocked discovery that "you've been reading *books*!"

There are, of course, universities where psychology and the acquisition of interview techniques is beginning to gain a foothold in medical courses. But even there these skills may be seen as means of acquiring power over patients and manipulating them effectively. A professor of obstetrics, describing the advances in the teaching of medical students in his own department, told me, "We have a film on how to deal with a difficult patient." (We are still awaiting, unfortunately, the film on how to deal with a difficult doctor.) He went on to explain some of the techniques of interviewing and counseling which were taught: "Eye contact is important," he said, and fixing me with an unwavering glare, added, "You will notice that I am making eye contact with *you* now."

As we have seen, the older woman may find that she is in a "high risk" category simply because of her age. For some obstetricians this classification includes all first-time mothers over thirty. Others tend to include in this category only women of thirty-five and older. A few believe that it should include women having first babies at twenty-eight. Different terms are used to describe the women. "Elderly primigravida" is one, which, as one woman said, "made me feel very long in the tooth." A woman who was five feet tall was very alarmed at being categorized as an "elderly *dwarf* primigravida." A "gravida" is simply a pregnant woman. So a "multigravida" is one who has had previous pregnancies. If you are pregnant but have had two miscarriages you are a "gravida"! The other term is "parity" to describe the number of previous pregnancies which have gone through to twenty-eight weeks or after. If you are "para 3" you have had three births. If you are "para 3 + 1" you have had three births and one miscarriage. Multiple births and miscarriages are counted as one in this system of reckoning. A "nulliparous" woman is one who is having her first pregnancy, though the terms "primagravida" or "primipara" are often used loosely instead.

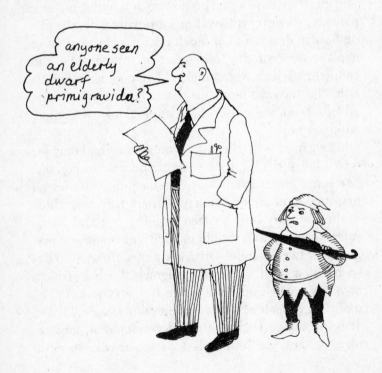

Doctors

Perinatal Mortality

Statistically, risks to the baby are higher to women giving birth over thirty than for those in their twenties. Under twenty the risks are also higher. The perinatal mortality rate (PMR) is a record of deaths of babies at birth or in the week following. The figure is given as a proportion of 1000 births. In the United States, the PMR is now about 12 per 1000. This is a crude figure, however, because it does not tell us anything about the quality of life of the babies who live or about the mothers who are most likely to have babies who live or about those who are most likely to have babies who die. Age is only one factor associated with perinatal mortality. It is clear that perinatal mortality reflects poverty. It stems from all the things we associate with social disadvantage: lack of education, poor housing, overcrowding, inadequate nutrition, stress, environmental poisons, and perhaps also simply from not being able to operate in "the system"—being powerless and unable even to claim social security benefits.

It is difficult to isolate these variables because being poor brings with it many other disadvantages for the fetus. Smoking in pregnancy is more common. Some eight deaths of every 1000 births might be avoided if women did not smoke when pregnant, and many more babies would arrive with better birth weights. Congenital malformations such as spina bifida, including those which are incompatible with life, are also more frequent at the bottom of the social scale, and these alone account for twenty-two percent of perinatal deaths. Seventy percent of babies who die do so because they are born prematurely. Here again there is an association with social class. The higher the social class, the lower the percentage of preterm births. The poor may live in heavily built-up inner-city areas, where lead from car exhausts pollutes the air. If a woman is at the bottom of the social scale she is more likely to get pregnant while still in her teens, and some women who cannot cope with contraception or whose partners are unwilling to, go on having babies when they are themselves in poor health. There is also a continuum of disadvantage; though individuals break out of the pattern, it tends to be passed on from parents to children. There is mounting evidence that it is important that a woman has good nutrition, not only during pregnancy, but before. This reflects the social-class culture in which she lives and perhaps also that in which she was reared. Her nutrition while she was growing up may be another factor in the equation, and perhaps even her own parents' nutrition.

The upshot of all this is that if you are reading this page the statistics of highest risk, stemming from poor social conditions, do not apply to you. If you are willing to abort a deformed fetus, having had AFP testing and, if it is advised, amniocentesis, any risk is still further reduced. In good health yourself and with a straightforward pregnancy in which no special risk factors are detected, you can expect a normal labor and a healthy baby. No one can guarantee this, but generalizations that older mothers always have difficult births, that an older woman's baby after a normal pregnancy is at greater risk, or that older mothers are less successful at breastfeeding are all untrue.

Doctors

It is difficult to measure pain or guess whether labor is likely to be more (or less) painful because of your age, because so much depends on your attitude of mind and whether you feel that pain is *attacking* you or working *for* you. This in itself is influenced by the environment in which birth takes place, by psychological factors such as whether or not you feel cherished and emotionally supported, and by such things as tiredness or exhaustion and conflicting emotions about what is happening. All these affect the perception of pain. One woman, who actually delivered in the bath at home, comfortably lapped in warm water, commented: "I do not want to give the impression that it was all dreamlike pleasure. Obviously if it had not been for the birth of our baby, the same sensations would have been painful. Only the love and the joy transformed the contractions into a 'labor' rather than a 'pain.'"

Induced Labor

Some obstetricians have a policy of inducing labor, that is, starting it artificially, in all their patients over a certain age. A doctor will sometimes tell the woman in early pregnancy, "I won't let you go past your due date at your age," or tell her to come into the hospital a week or two weeks *before* she is due, to be induced. Unless you have a *medical* condition, the most common of which is diabetes, which means that labor should be started early, an obstetrician cannot possibly tell whether you can be induced with safety to your baby while you are still in the first half of pregnancy. Even with modern methods of estimating gestation such as serial ultrasound, mistakes can be made about the age of the fetus, and occasionaly babies are delivered before they are ready for life, with consequent breathing problems.

The length of pregnancy is assumed to be 280 days or forty weeks, often regardless of the length of the menstrual cycle. When periods have been irregular it is especially difficult to know when ovulation occurred. Thirty percent of babies are delivered before the estimated date and seventy percent after that date. Most pregnancies last anywhere between thirty-eight and forty-two weeks, though ninety percent of births take place within ten days of the due date. Your age is an insufficient reason for inducing labor.

Inductions should be performed only after you have discussed the reasons for it, had time to think about it, been told exactly what happens, and given your consent. It is easier for you to consider the matter if you are out of the hospital, in your normal surroundings. Some doctors expect patients to agree on the spot, or else send them into an adjoining room for a few minutes to make up their minds. You can say, "I'd like more time to think about this, and I don't think I can let you know before next Tuesday," or "I want time to talk this over with my husband," though the doctor may then ask, "Is your husband an obstetrician?" and if you say no, say, "Well, how can he possibly help you decide, then?" (which is what happened to one woman of thirty-six).

Your childbirth educator may be a good person with whom to discuss possible induction. She knows what happens and will probably also know which obstetricians perform it most readily, and if they tend to pressure their patients into it or frequently suggest that the baby will die if the induction does not go ahead. Some obstetricians regularly subject their patients to a form of emotional blackmail. Women say that they are asked, "Are you prepared to accept responsibility if your baby dies?" or "You do realize you are risking your baby's life, do you?"

If an expectant mother tries to discuss episiotomy, a cut made to enlarge the birth outlet, some obstetricians may make her feel accused of deliberately intending to injure her baby by making the birth difficult for it, and threatened with postnatal frigidity and the consequent breakdown of her marriage and by prolapse later in life unless she agrees to one. These obstetricians genuinely believe that their way is better than nature's and can offer improved and, what Sir John Dewhurst, former President of the Royal College of Gynecologists and Obstetricians in Britain, calls "enhanced" childbirth. They are sincere and often deeply committed to their beliefs. When you discuss your treatment with them, bear this in mind.

Though it may be taken for granted that an older woman needs an episiotomy, understanding of the way a woman's body functions in childbirth and support from her attendants to push spontaneously, without commands or coaxing, only as much as and when *she* wants to, often enables her to give birth without one. It is no wonder that women tear or require an episiotomy when they are urged to hold their breath and ordered to push as long and as hard as they are able. Under these conditions even emptying our bowels would also be painful and traumatic. Moreover, lying or sitting positions put more strain on the perineum. Side-lying or upright positions, such as crouching, kneeling, squatting forward, standing, or being on all fours, all reduce stress on the perineum and distribute pressure more evenly on the tissues surrounding the vagina.

If it is your first baby, the second stage may take longer than it would have done when you were younger because the head needs to press down gradually through layers of tissue, opening them out rather like a fan-pleated skirt, and it is the first time you will have opened up this wide. It is often assumed that a first-time older mother has tissues that are inflexible, without the "give" of younger tissues. But there have been no studies published on this, and since we know that tissue flexibility is affected by general health and by diet, it may be that an older woman in good health and on a balanced diet can have tissues that are in better condition than those of a younger woman in poor health who keeps going on "junk" food. An older woman who pays particular attention to perineal well-being, with pelvic-floor exercises performed not just at exercise sessions but as movements throughout the day, and who, perhaps, also uses oil to massage her perineum regularly and help her get the feeling of "giving," is preparing herself in the best way for delivery without the need of episiotomy. Since this operation is performed as routine by many physicians, however, it is important to speak to your doctor about it in advance. Tell him that you want to deliver without episiotomy, if possible, and ask him to help you achieve this.

Though your childbirth educator can probably give

you information, she is usually torn between giving you facts so that you can decide for yourself and making things as easy and comfortable as possible for you so that whatever happens you are able to adapt to labor. She may say to herself, "If this woman is going to have an induced labor anyway, I can help her accept it psychologically and reassure her about what happens." And she is quite right if she tells you that some women have very happy, straightforward induced labors. On the other hand, many do not. Though techniques of induction have improved in most hospitals since 1978, the date of my own study of women's experiences of induction,[3] research then revealed that women being induced needed far more painkillers. Ninety-five percent of women who had attended National Childbirth Trust prenatal classes had drugs for pain relief when labor was induced. Women who go to classes often hope to manage without drugs as far as possible. When labor was not induced, fifty percent of women managed without them. Those women who had already had babies with a noninduced labor were asked to compare the induced labor with the previous labor which was not induced. Usually second births are easier than the first. The majority of these women said that the second birth was *more* painful.

The babies did not do so well either, though more babies of induced labors were probably at risk for other reasons. A much larger proportion of newborns were separated from their mothers because they were put in the special care nursery. These babies were unlikely all to have been ill, since policy used to be to put every baby delivered after a difficult labor under the watchful eyes of the special care nurse just in case. Since the publication of the work of Klaus and Kennell on bonding[4] this policy has been changed in many hospitals.

Because of the analgesics the mothers had taken there was also another kind of separation. Many women experienced a pharmacological separation from their babies, whom they could not hold because they felt too "woozy" or could not see because they fell asleep. This separation severely affected the first meeting between mother and baby immediately following delivery and for several hours afterward. It also affected breastfeeding, since the time when the baby can most naturally and easily go to the mother's breast after birth was missed. Many of the babies were knocked out by the drugs the mother had taken. This was usually Demerol or Demerol in combination with other drugs.

Once labor is induced and the bag of waters has been ruptured, there is no way back. The obstetrician is committed to getting you delivered within twenty-four hours. To wait any longer than this increases the risk of infection. He has to be prepared, therefore, to engage in "active management" to keep to a timetable. Professor Ian Donald warns that "any intervention, however apparently trivial, carries with it the responsibilities for consequences . . ."[5] The decision to induce labor is as serious a one as a decision to perform a cesarean section. The rate of intravenous oxytocin can be stepped up to make the uterus work harder. This may cause more pain, so Demerol or an epidural anesthetic may be offered before this is done or shortly after. If the cervix fails to dilate or the baby reacts with type two dips in its heart rate (a slowing of the baby's heart after the end of a contraction), ones that persist after the contraction has ended, the obstetrician will be ready to intervene with cesarean section. If the cervix dilates but there is a holdup then, because the woman has an epidural and cannot feel how to push or is too doped or exhausted to do so, delivery can be by forceps, or sometimes by vacuum extractor. Induced labors are more likely to finish with forceps[6] or cesarean[7] deliveries.

Failed Induction

An induction that ends in a cesarean section is a *failed* induction. Two percent upward of all inductions end in a cesarean. Professor Donald says: "No method of induction is both absolutely certain and safe."[8] In Britain induction was most in vogue in the early seventies. Then nearly forty percent of all labors were induced. The rate has fallen steadily since then, largely because it has been discovered that high induction rates do not save babies' lives. But there is still wide variation between different hospitals and even inside the same hospital between different physicians. You can ask the obstetrician the induction rate in his group. If it is below about fifteen percent, listen with great care to his explanation of why you need to be induced because he will have very good reasons. If it is over twenty-five percent, some labors are probably being induced unnecessarily. Between these two figures there is a gray area, because hospitals in different parts of the country care for women from widely varying backgrounds, and high-risk women from poor social backgrounds *may* benefit from a greater proportion of induced labors than women who have no known risk factors. In fact, studies reveal that women from lower social classes get *less* intervention than middle-class women."[9]

It is widely believed that since the induction "scare" of the seventies induction rates have plummeted. This is not so. And even where fewer inductions are done, acceleration of labors that have already started is common. This practice too has its risks, which are much the same as those of induction. Some obstetricians believe that it is right to manage actively the labors of all first-time mothers over thirty or thirty-five. It is more difficult to resist an intravenous drip of synthetic oxytocin once you are already in the hospital and in bed. But no intervention should take place unless you have it explained to you and you have agreed to it. In practice, once a patient has been told about a procedure in however rudimentary a way ("I'm going to give you a bit of help now" or "I'm just going to give you a little prick"—one woman, usually refined, exclaimed, "I don't care whether it is big or little. I don't want it!"), it is taken that she has understood and accepted the intervention. So you have to be quick to say, "No, thank you" or "Hold on! I'd like to discuss this."

Induction should be done in only two circumstances: when the baby is obviously safer out than in because the intrauterine environment is poor; and when the mother's health is going to suffer severely if the pregnancy continues. The cervix should be ripe, and if it is not, a failed induction is quite likely. Measures used to ripen the cervix include nipple stimulation for several days and, in some centers, prostaglandin suppositories placed in the cervix. The latter technique is being used experimentally in the United States and is in wide use in Britain. Sometimes oxytocin is unnecessary, as labor proceeds with prostaglandin or breast stimulation alone. This is much more comfortable for the mother and may allow labor to progress more normally because she can be up and about.

If you are induced, do not expect labor to be rapid. It can be long and drawn-out, and the so-called latent phase before there is effective dilation of the cervix may be prolonged.

Similarly, if a cesarean section is recommended, though the news comes as a shock, take time to discuss the pros and cons with your doctor. It may be that a trial of labor, with everything ready for a cesarean section if necessary, is a better idea. In many cases no one knows for sure what a uterus can do until contractions have gotten under way. If it proves to be a cesarean after all, consider the possibility of one with epidural anesthesia. This enables you to awake when your baby is born and aware of everything that is going on. Abby, a new mother, said it was "fantastic!"

> They erected a green curtain across my tummy so I couldn't see. I felt no pain, only pressure. Then as soon as they delivered the baby they lowered the curtain and gave her to me. I fell in love with her straight away. Bill then came in and I was stitched up . . . We were lost in wonder over our new daughter.

In many hospitals fathers are now able to be present at a cesarean under epidural, and this is worth asking for if you think you would both enjoy it. If an obstetrician has not had a father there before, he may find it helpful and reassuring to meet your man beforehand and may be willing to try it as an experiment with someone he already knows.

Self-Doubt

Seeds of self-doubt are sometimes sown in an older woman's mind during pregnancy inadvertently by other people's remarks. You laugh them off at the time but in the middle of the night they sprout. One woman of thirty-eight said that pregnant teenagers in the hospital were "aghast" when they learned her age and exclaimed, "You're old enough to be my mother!" and "My God! You never imagine *teachers* having *babies*!" Older mothers often mention remarks made at the clinic. "You're a bit old for this sort of thing, aren't you?" or "We'll have to keep an eye on you." One woman was lying on the examination table with her lower half exposed when the doctor swept in, followed by a retinue of students, notebooks poised. "Ah," exclaimed the great man, "here we have the perfect example of an elderly primigravida!" "And a *talking* elderly primigravida too!" said the patient, raising her head.

In spite of feeling vulnerable and at a disadvantage with her pants down, the woman over thirty really does have more of a chance of getting the doors of communication open with the doctors, even if they often need a bit of a shove. She may be of the same age and social class as those caring for her, so they have that in common, or the doctor may be younger so that she does not feel in awe of him.

A sense of humor helps, if only because the woman who insists on knowing what is to be done to her and why is readily labeled as "anxious," "neurotic," or "difficult," and this may be written into her notes. If you can be firm and persistent but at the same time keep a light touch, you give yourself more chance of genuine "rapport." If you have a male partner, taking him with you to meet the obstetrician means that he not only appreciates what you go through at your pre-natal visits but can ask questions too. It may also put the obstetrician more at ease, as some hospital doctors do not like talking to women and find it much simpler to talk "man to man." If you do this, you have to be sure that the two will not start colluding together, how-ever, and making decisions *for* you. Get as much in-formation as you can, first of all; talk through together in advance the things that matter most to you and make notes of priorities. You might even try acting through a hypothetical discussion, taking turns playing the part of the obstetrician. If the answer to a question is un-convincing, how are you going to follow it up? Re-member that you do not have to come to any snap decisions. Unless there is a dire emergency, you can always take time to think things through. Just say, "I'd like time to think about that."

Talk with your doctor as a human being, not as an authoritarian professional in a white coat. (Think of him in his pajamas.) And bear in mind that most ob-stetricians are rushed, overworked, and under great pressure, because they see far too many patients in too

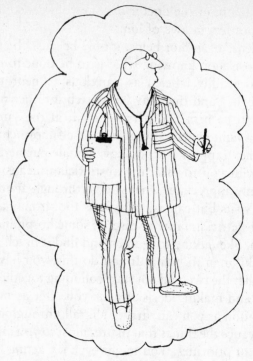

Think of your doctor in his pajamas

short a time. This does not mean that you should not take time to talk because you are aware of the other patients waiting (though that is a natural reaction) but that you think ahead to what you want to say, use the interview constructively, and *thank* him for giving the time. Sheer pressure of numbers sometimes means that you have to put off a discussion until the next visit. Some doctors spend on average only two minutes with each patient. Explain that this discussion is important to you and make at least an unofficial appointment for it. If you cannot get anyone to make time for you, write a letter to the obstetrician. Once something is in the files it tends to be noticed, if only because it is open to other people's perusal too.

Some of the problems older mothers encounter in pregnancy and labor result from the obstetrician's concern about them and from too much doctoring rather than from any inherent condition. Pregnancy is seen primarily not as a natural physiological state but as a hazardous process. Judith Lumley, a lecturer in obstetrics in Australia, puts it this way:

> The distinction between normal and abnormal pregnancy has become blurred. Some doctors reject the "normal" as inappropriate, and classify all pregnant women as low risk, medium risk or high risk patients. Normality becomes an accolade, to be bestowed after the event on the few women who pass through pregnancy and birth without deviating from the physiological ideal at any point.[10]

In this the older pregnant woman, especially one having a baby for the first time, has all the odds stacked against her. Obstetric and midwifery textbooks sometimes discuss her as if she had one foot in the grave, with increased chances of uterine fibroids, miscarriage, hypertension, premature labor, long, dysfunctional labor, forceps delivery, and cesarean sjection. It is understandable that the doctor who does not have much experience of the normal, healthy older pregnant woman may become anxious and then convey this anxiety to his patient. When a woman's blood pressure goes up, for example, this may be a direct result of a proliferation of investigations that threaten confidence, warnings from doctors, and stressful prenatal appointments. The woman goes in feeling happy and fit and comes out feeling reproductively incompetent and sick with fear, frustration, and, often, suppressed anger. It would be surprising if this did *not* have an effect on her blood pressure.

Keeping Calm

It may help to build some calm into your daily life: Yoga, meditation, relaxation or a space for slow full breathing, or simply luxuriating in a leisurely bath in a darkened room. Finding a way to express what you feel is also vital. Your anger is legitimate and it can help to cry, shout, or bash the pillows. Most women try to go on as if nothing had happened and to be "reasonable," thus giving implicit acceptance to the assumption that anything can be required of a woman *for the sake of her baby*. Objecting to the way you are being treated in the prenatal clinic seems selfish since it is all being done for your baby.

Some older women have relatively good experiences with prenatal clinics and hospital care, especially those who have careers in the health services. They feel they are on familiar ground and may know those caring for them. Others enjoy being part of the workings of an efficiently run institution and feel secure and confident with the application of modern technology to the business of childbirth. Fran says that her "present idea of heaven would be to spend a week in the hospital, *enjoying* anonymity, gloriously free from domestic demands and the company of my (albeit loving) family." With a sideswipe at my own views she adds: "Some women are not so Luddite as to be thrown into hysteria at the sight of gleaming machinery, or so childlike as to need to depend on Daddy the Doctor or Mommy the Midwife." Even she, however, describes one incident in her happy hospital experience in which she felt completely depersonalized. She had been pushed out of the delivery room on a trolley and was going up to the ward in an elevator, surrounded by porters and nurses:

> They were joking about their weekend dates and I wondered if it would be rude to join in the conversation. But it became clear to me that it wasn't expected. I was simply a body in transit.

It takes an effort of will and imagination to move on from that situation to accept that doctors, midwives, and nurses can be collaborators rather than powerful authority figures appropriating from us the responsibility for the outcome of the pregnancy. Though a distorted medical perspective often implies that statistics ought to rule our lives, personal experience tells us that such views of life are untenable. The value we attach to particular events and qualities of relationships must also affect the decisions we make. If we thought only in terms of statistics and of reducing the perinatal mortality by one more decimal point, no matter what effect this had on human emotions and values, we could make it a matter of public policy to detect all multiple pregnancies by ultrasound and abort them immediately. This would prevent 800 deaths each year in England and Wales alone. That we do not do so shows that values do not depend on mere arithmetic. Even doctors most passionately concerned about perinatal mortality statistics have not proposed this solution. Nor can we ever have *complete* safety in childbirth. Expecting a baby to be perfect if you do all the right things and have every available investigation sets an impossibly high and unrealistic standard. As more and more tests for fetal well-being are developed, a situation may develop in which the older expectant mother could spend much of her time undergoing investigative procedures of one kind or another. The decision as to how much to probe and investigate is not a medical matter in the long run, but has to do with the quality of life and how much intervention we are prepared to tolerate for the sake of more knowledge. The pursuit of perfection in human reproduction is a mirage.

Ross Mitchell of the Department of Child Health at Dundee University expresses it this way:

In human reproduction, the analogy of the production line or conveyor belt is inappropriate: it implies a uniform, repeatable, and flawless standard of product, anything less than this being instantly and rightly rejected. In laying too great emphasis on the goal of faultless excellence, we may have done a misservice to some children and their parents. Every person is the result of many interacting influences, some beneficial and others inimical to development. The mother's anxious scrutiny of her new baby to assure herself that he is unblemished and her overreaction to the slightest deviation from an ideal norm are intensified by the tacit professional assumption that perfection is the yardstick.[11]

6

◆

Life After
the Baby Comes

When you are still pregnant it is very difficult to summon the imaginative energy to think about how things may be after the baby comes. Discussions about how you might feel, for instance, seem purely academic. The birth is the all-important challenge. Yet for many women that fourth trimester of pregnancy, the three months after the birth, its delights and difficulties, are more exciting, exhausting, and deeply satisfying than even the birth itself. You are bucketed out of a peak emotional experience straight into an activity and commitment that keeps you at full speed almost twenty-four hours of every day.

First-time older mothers say:

The most devastating thing is that once the child is born it is a total stranger. You have some idea of the times it will wake and sleep from the times it has been kicking you to bits, but otherwise you know nothing about it. This is frightening.

I felt I was a feeding and changing machine. The constant physical and emotional involvement with a dependent small human being was such a contrast to my previous life (as a librarian in an academic library). I realized how unprepared I was. Watching a public health nurse bathe a doll is a far cry from the real thing.

I had awful depression on the third day. Difficult because Robert (my husband) was still physically and emotionally exhausted. He's not used to feeling so much so intensely. We yelled at each other and I cried and wanted to die—about what we're going to eat for dinner, for goodness sake! The midwife was worried and asked her relief to come in next day—to find me up and about singing and washing diapers.

Having been a teacher used to dealing with about thirty-five children, I thought I'd find a baby a piece of cake. Although I was on a "high," I still found those first six weeks totally exhausting. I fell in love with my daughter from the first second I saw her. It really was like being in love. Every time I woke up I'd be overwhelmed with excitement, yes, even at three in the morning, I loved being with her, near her, touching her, kissing her, looking at her, and thinking constantly of her. ╱

The responsibility for this new life can be frightening. A woman who has been anxiously trying to fit the whole business of having a baby and rearing it into her own well-organized life-style may sometimes feel as if the ground has opened beneath her. The conflict be-

Birth Over Thirty

tween her career goals, her wants and the demands of her own ego, and the overwhelming pull of the baby's needs may produce grotesque and disturbing fantasies, both nighttime dreams and daytime mind-images that have the quality of hallucinations. A woman who had taken steps to be sterilized before she decided she wanted to have a baby was deeply troubled by the sense of her power to avoid pregnancy. It was as if she were the bad queen or the wicked witch of the story books:

> Every night since I came home from the hospital I have woken up not knowing where she is, thinking that she's in the bed, or believing that she's been squashed or suffocated. Sometimes the disturbance is quite mild and John tells me that she's in her room. At the other extreme, I have woken up crying out and desperately searching for her under the pillows.

There is also the astonishing reality of the baby, not just a package but a person. Many women feel the wave of passionate love that enthralls them is so intense that it makes it difficult to cope in the "real" world, with its lunch and supper times, daily routines, dealing with visitors, the questions people ask, and the demands of other human relations and people's expectations of you. Sylvia Plath vividly suggests the strength of this complete giving of oneself to the baby in her poem "Three Women."[1]

> What did my fingers do before they held him?
> What did my heart do with its love?
> I have never seen a thing so dear.
> His lids are like the lilac-flower

Life After the Baby Comes

And soft as a moth, his breath.
I shall not let go.

If you have already had a baby, even ten years ago, you know all about this and can smile in the recollection; you think back to the feelings of utter incompetence, perhaps, the awful self-doubts, the panic, the emotional swings, the sweetness as the baby lay sleeping peacefully, the awesome responsibility of protecting and caring for this new life, the firmness of the rounded limbs against your body, the heaviness of the head as a feeding finishes in utter content, the fine down on the skin, and the scent of warm peaches.

A Whetted Appetite

Women having another baby after a long space, though they may feel aghast at what they have done, and though at the beginning of pregnancy they may be resentful about being, as one woman said, "put back firmly in the home" and "trapped," look forward to these things with whetted appetite. They know it will be crazy and chaotic, but it is going to be fun! It is not just a question of the baby "keeping you young," either; it may feel once the baby is really there as if the choice is between rejuvenation and collapse.

The mother of a "surprise" baby often feels a special passionate closeness to the child. One said that this was "almost psychic." "Perhaps," she added, "we have to fight for their entry into this world that much more and the fight has provided the bond." She had faced the idea of abortion and after a struggle had decided firmly against it, in the face of other people's advice. One battle for this particular woman was against the horrified disapproval of her own mother, who would not speak to her for six months. Many women also feel that the hurdles of tests through which they go during pregnancy are also like part of a long struggle to have the baby.

When the older woman compares her experience with the late-born baby with how she was as a mother with earlier children, she always says how much more relaxed, confident, and at ease she is this time round. Women having a second family have a different time scale from even those older mothers who are having their first-born children, and say they spend time with the baby because everything else seems relatively un-important. "I know that time passes all too quickly when children are small," remarks one mother, pre-viously in educational research, "and that these early years are crucial for future learning, social behavior, and exploration." The experienced mother also realizes that problems that seem insurmountable at the time all pass before long. One who felt "cloistered" with her baby during feeding times that went on and on and on remembered that this stage was a temporary one, and reflected that she needed this time to get to know her baby properly and to protect herself from outside stresses.

For the first-time mother over thirty the initial chal-lenges appear rather different. Looking ahead to the enforced change of role, the excitement is mixed with anxiety, not just about coping, but about what the baby's arrival will do to her as a person. For a time it is delightful not to have to rush out and be "bright and interesting," but even while she basks in this satisfaction there may be stirrings of restlessness. This is intensified if the baby is at first unwanted. As one woman, commenting on the distress she experienced after the birth of her baby, said:

> I lost my personal space. My overriding preoccupation is how I am going to get back to work. At first I thought I'd probably have to give up work and felt very resentful of the baby. It was a tremendous upheaval to discover I was pregnant. I have a fantastic physician, and he made a lot of time to talk so that I didn't bottle this up inside. I decided, Yes, I do want to have the baby. Now I'm anxious about how we are going to get along. Will we like each other? How are we going to sort this one out together?

Her opportunity to talk freely with her physician helped her move out of concern solely with what the birth of the baby was going to do to *her* to a concern about her relationship with this new person. Without the opportunity to talk, that progression might have been delayed until well after the baby came.

A Career Crisis

Having a baby after thirty provokes a career crisis that the older mother often realizes may never be resolved. One woman, completely committed to her career and unwilling to take time out from it, said her mind was only set at rest when her obstetrician said, "Right! I promise to keep you working as long as I can and to get you back to work as soon as possible after." Many women are far less sure that this is what they want. They do not know whether they will want to go back to work, or if they intend to do so, how soon they and the baby will be ready for this. Shall it be job, baby, or job and baby? The law is now that a woman cannot be dismissed from her job because of pregnancy. The decision as to whether, in fact, you want to return is yours, and you can change your mind at any time. If you say when you leave that you do not want to return, however, you are closing the door on the options open to you. If you work only part-time or have not been in the same employment for very long, you may not be entitled to maternity leave.

A pregnant woman may be very uncertain of what her own feelings are going to be after the baby arrives, and perhaps does not trust that she is ever going to fall in love with her baby.

"Your career is about to take off or is already well established," Tricia explained. "For me it was the problem of when to break and that if I did have two or three years out it would be difficult to get back in."

Virginia said she planned to do a postgraduate degree to "keep her mind awake" and was afraid that having a baby would fuddle her brain unless she took determined steps to develop new career skills.

Financial problems may loom large, not because of an overall shortage of money but because a woman in her thirties is usually earning more than she did ten years before and the disappearance of one partner's salary makes a dramatic difference. She is often anxious

Life After the Baby Comes

about the loss of independence and freedom that come from having her own income:

> Thinking of being financially dependent on my husband upsets me. I've been independent for so long. I feel trapped by the thought that I have to ask for money for the everyday things of life, having to say, "Please, can I have $20.00 because I can't get through this month?" or "Would you mind paying the milk bill?"

A woman who says she is "lucky" because she works two hours a day at home designing children's clothes says that without this and her own money she might feel frustrated. The dependence that is being fought against is more than economic. For many women it expresses anxiety about a loss of selfhood.

The fear is that you are somehow going to be sucked in by baby care, your brain will turn vegetable, and you will become "just a mother." A woman to whom children are stuck like "barnacles encrusting a ship and limpets clinging to a rock" is the awful image summoned up by Margaret Atwood in *The Edible Woman*.[2] For the committed feminist there is the inherent threat that she has "sold out" to motherhood and to a role stereotype that legitimizes the social inferiority of women. One woman said that her feminist friends "are upset at my loss of independence, and opting out."

First-time mothers look very carefully at their friends and relations who have small children. They watch them with all the vigilance and concentration of an ethologist observing a pack of orangutans. And they tend to come away highly critical of what they see.

111

Birth Over Thirty

Total Devotion

A group of pregnant women, all having first babies in their thirties, were discussing the kind of mother they hoped to be. They were all anxious about devoting themselves entirely to a baby.

"I know a couple who haven't been out to dinner with each other for eighteen months," Maureen said.

"I know," said another, "it's the same with friends of ours. But it's a very awkward baby. It won't sleep for longer than three hours and she is just so tired."

"I get rather cross at the relish with which other women say, 'Oh, you won't have a minute to yourself, you won't have time to read a book.' " Julia protested. "They seem to *enjoy* saying this. I just cannot imagine not having time to read or to write a letter. I can't imagine being so tired. It makes me very depressed."

"From some of the things people say," Jan exclaimed, "I get the feeling that I'm expected to metamorphize into a completely different person. Two friends who are doctors and who were at the peaks of their careers said, 'It's wonderful to vegetate at home.' I don't think it will be. I have a fear that something *biological* will happen to me."

Another woman remarked that even during her pregnancy friends seem to be distancing themselves. "It's almost as if being pregnant is supposed to affect your decision making and therefore your opinions are not worth listening to (though your husband's are)."

The contrast between these anxieties and the surge of emotion that comes with being a new mother is startling. The woman no longer seems to be protecting herself in the same way. Joan, a nurse for twenty years who had her first baby at thirty-eight, said she feared that she had thrown away her last vestige of independence forever when she became pregnant. She went on from there to describe the emotional journey into motherhood.

After a difficult and painful seventeen-hour labor she had a forceps delivery and her baby was taken immediately to the intensive care nursery.

> I confess I was relieved not to have to look after him the first night as I was deeply shocked by all the pain. But during the days that followed I was filled with pure delight at this little person who I found hard to believe was really mine. I appreciate that having babies is old hat to most people and there is nothing unique about my experience, but the feelings that came to me so unexpectedly were ones of overwhelming emotion for which I felt I had been ill-prepared. Sometimes I was torn apart by the thought that something might happen to the baby. He means much more to me than I had imagined.

The emotions that flood in as the baby is lifted out of your body are often unexpected and seem to have no connection with more conventional ideas of love. Some older women who have had no contact with small babies and have read about the importance of bonding are anxious that they will not be able to respond with appropriate emotions at delivery and that those present will criticize them for their inability to bond. In fact, for any mother there is often a phase of stunned astonishment, an interval when she needs time to find herself again. Moira expressed this when she said:

> The head oozed out and then the shoulders were eased through. He came resembling a wee lizard; all my emotions were frozen in a void with this beautiful yet very ugly creature lying on my tummy. Then Tony [her husband] told us how clever we were, which gave the moment warm snowflakes.

The first-time mother, whatever her age, often is rather frightened of her child at first. "I thought she was lovely," one woman said, "but was scared and lived in a fog of worry and uncertainty until she was six weeks old. Then the fog cleared miraculously and there we were the three of us intact."

Jan was right, of course, when she suspected that the change which takes place is at least partly biological. The woman at term is primed physiologically and psychologically in readiness of motherhood. The release of hormones into her bloodstream during and following labor (the rush of oxytocin that is in a way still incompletely understood) is linked with uterine contractions, working to open the cervix and press the baby down the birth canal. This subsequently contracts the uterus to expel the placenta and mold it back into its former shape, and drives her forward emotionally, too. She is carried on a wave of powerful emotions, a passion that is for many women intensely sexual in its pain and pleasure. Dr. Michel Odent of Pithiviers (author of *Birth Reborn,* Pantheon, 1984) describes oxytocin as "the happiness hormone," released only when the woman feels she can trust herself and her body. This and other hormones flood her bloodstream during the days following birth, making her emotionally labile, vulnerable, and above all, responsive.

This acute physiological link with the baby lasts for many women for about six weeks and for some much longer. It corresponds to the period of "primary maternal preoccupation" described by Donald Winnicott, the pediatrician and psychotherapist, though the term does nothing to convey the powerful "gut feelings" and the almost animal nature of the bond between the mother and her newborn. It has clearly been important to the survival of the species.

Selfless Giving

The new mother is often enormously surprised to discover her capacity for selfless giving and a patience far beyond her expectations. She is in partnership with her baby, sending out signals involving touch, scent, the rhythm of her breathing and heartbeats; her eyes are turned toward the baby and her voice raised to a higher than usual pitch, as she speaks in a pattern of five- to fifteen-second intervals and quite unconsciously repeats the phrases with a strong beat that have meaning for all babies and in all languages.

Apparently casual, random behavior is, in fact, perfectly adjusted to the needs and attention span of this new baby. The mother leans forward so that she is face to face with her baby and about a forearm's length away, the distance at which the child can most easily focus on her shining eyes and mobile mouth, and the one at which a baby is naturally held when breast-feeding. She raises her eyebrows quite spontaneously and begins to talk. The baby's attention is caught by the movement. She smiles and the relief planes of her face are increased. In a questioning tone of voice, re-iterating simple syllables, she starts to "rev up" the baby, exaggerating her facial expression, perhaps grimacing, and she may do that over and over again, like an angler throwing a line. At last the baby catches on and gets excited. Eyes light up; the lips form a shape; there may be a little gurgle or coo of pleasure. The relationship between mother and baby is a going concern!

Far from being a passive little bundle, the newborn baby seeks stimuli, explores, and starts out on a new adventure. The child, too, is sending out signals and plays an active role in this partnership. He gazes at his mother's forehead and she hovers nearer, trying to catch his eyes. At last she gets his attention, and in the early days for a brief time only the two begin a conversation together, until the baby gets bored with it and attention wanders. The anxious mother continues to hover and try to stimulate the baby to respond. The relaxed one releases the baby to turn to something else of interest or to be fairly passive until the next burst of conversation between them. It is as if the two are learning a dance together. When the mother is anxious or de-pressed, or the baby is suffering the effects of pain-relieving drugs received from her bloodstream during labor, or has a headache from a difficult birth, it takes longer for them to learn that dance of interaction. But it is astonishing how many mothers and babies, even though the mother feels she has no "maternal instincts" or has worried that she will be "tied down" by a baby or that her "mind will rot," start to enjoy each other.

They both have the advantage of much more primitive preverbal signals too than we are inclined to acknowledge in adult life. Smell is one of them. Many new mothers comment on the delicious scent of their babies. The baby, for her part, responds to the mother's smell. Dr. Aidan MacFarlane, an Oxford pediatrician, has shown how even five-day-old babies prefer a breast-pad that has been against their own mother's breast to one worn by a strange mother. The maternal scent is intensified by heat produced in the mother's breasts as she responds to her baby's cry. It is not only the smell of milk but a scent emanating from her skin that the baby senses. This is partly because the woman who has recently delivered is very warm and during the first days after birth perspires freely, losing the fluid that was retained in her tissues in the last weeks of pregnancy. I do not know of anything that has ever been written about the smell of puerperal blood. We usually treat it as merely a messy waste-product, an aftermath of childbirth. But it has a strong, clinging, and exciting smell that is in some ways intensely sexual. The baby cannot fail to be aware of this afterbirth blood scent. As the baby sucks at the breast, oxytocin makes the uterus contract further and more blood is squeezed out, sometimes (especially early in the morning, after lying down for some hours) in heavy velvet clots.

For a woman who has not yet had her baby this may seem revolting. But with birth come strange new pleasures, deep below the ground of our conscious being and having nothing to do with the more conventional pleasures of having a baby. It is as well to have a mind open to them, too.

Eager to Learn

At the same time a good deal of more obvious cerebral activity is taking place. If you watch carefully you can see that the baby is eager and quick to learn. Wait till she is in a quiet, alert state, comfortable with her body, not hungry, but wide awake and staring at you. Then stick out your tongue. The chances are that after a few false starts there will be a flicker of movement from the baby's mouth and she, too, will try to put out her tongue. After a few days of this game, done only when

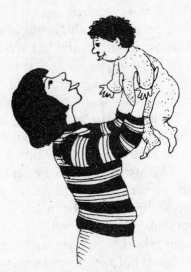

Then stick out your tongue . . .

the baby is happy and attentive, she will mimic you effectively. It is the beginning of a great game. It is on such copying that the learning of language and the more general acquisition of culture is based in each society. Long before speech the patterns of mouth movements and even facial expressions are already set.

It is important to let the baby set the pace. The overstimulated baby, entertained too vigorously by an adult who wants to prove that he or she can be successful, turns away and gazes hard at something else, ignoring the brash stimulus and making the intruder feel rejected. If this happens too often a parent can feel like a failure. Some babies enjoy more stimuli than others. You need to get to know your baby. If you act just according to the book, or set an educational scheme going that is insensitive to what your baby is telling you, the relationship is hampered from the start.

While the trigger for all this is a biological one, important in creating the bonds of the family and the handing on of culture in all human communities, the specific scene is that offered by the environment in which the mother first meets and begins to get to know her baby. For most women in the Western world nowadays, this is a hospital. The atmosphere provided in that setting can help or inhibit bonding. This atmosphere is only indirectly created by curtains or furnishings. It is made by *people*.

The way the relationship starts is not entirely dependent on what is happening during the time following delivery. It is in part an outcome of everything that has happened to the mother in labor and while she was pregnant. She has not been merely a container for the

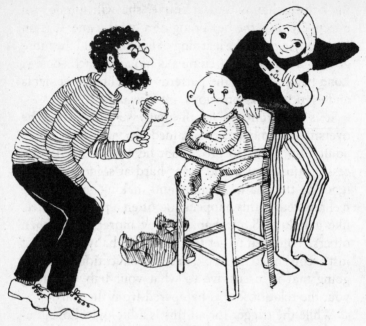

The overstimulated baby

fetus. What she feels about the act of birth and the care she is given, the way she is treated as a person, not just as a caretaker for the baby, affects her ability to relate to her child. When she feels cherished and among friends, free to act spontaneously without stopping to wonder whether she is doing the right thing or obeying the rules or reaching a set standard, she can most enjoy her baby.

With loving emotional support and in a relaxed atmosphere, the most unlikely woman starts out on motherhood with gusto. It is not a matter of doing the "right" thing; there is no right way to look after a

120

baby. It is more a matter of doing what you feel like doing and not getting self-conscious about it. Even if you do not get the chance to be yourself while you are still in the hospital and do not fall in love with your baby until after you come home, you need not feel that you have missed a limited opportunity that time and circumstances have gobbled up. In human relationships there are always, fortunately, second, third, and even fourth chances. Each of the anxious pregnant women who were discussing their fears of the future and their loss of self-esteem discovered that they were surprised at the pleasure they found in what one called "the exquisite beauty of captivity to a baby."

A Support Network

If you are expecting your first baby after thirty, it is a good idea to contact other women in the same age group who are having or have just had their babies. Your doctor or midwife may be able to help. Your prenatal teacher or the local childbirth education association certainly can. It is not only useful to get together beforehand to discuss the changes in your lives. It may also be helpful to have a support network afterward, and to know that there is someone you can ring who is tackling similar difficulties. Many childbirth education organizations have postnatal support groups. You can either use the existing structure or get something going yourself that is specifically for older first-time mothers.

It can take some courage to make new contacts after

the baby comes, and it may be difficult to get out to meet other people unless you have arranged things in advance. A new mother of forty, whose friends all had children in their teens, said it was a totally alien world to her, and it was not until she started taking her child to playgroup that she caught up with social contacts that otherwise would have passed her by.

> I meet these efficient twenty- to twenty-five-year-olds wisely discussing child management and nursery groups. For all my gray hairs I think it must be good to have this link with a much younger group. Perhaps it will keep me feeling younger, if I'm not worn out by the effort.

Ella went through a difficult time when her little daughter was three to six months old, a time when the novelty of having a baby has worn off and when most women find endlessly repeated tasks are beginning to get them down. With Ella it was particularly hard because Penny was awake most of the day, sleeping only four half-hour stretches:

> Unlike what the books say she was definitely *not* happy sitting in her bouncing chair and watching Mommy doing things. *She* wanted to be doing things and found it very frustrating that she couldn't. She therefore wanted my constant attention so we could "do" things together.

Ella felt she was "foundering in a sea of baby and wondering if I'd ever surface." She started shouting at her baby, and was then submerged in guilt. Her husband could not help, as he had just started making a new film and came home late each evening, emotionally and physically drained. She began to feel very lonely and to long for adult company:

> I met at my local clinic a mother who was part of the local postnatal support group. From then on I never looked back. I became involved with other mothers of similar interests and background (in their thirties, had careers, etc.). I had people to share my new experiences and difficulties with, and we gave each other support.

She started helping other mothers who were still at a stage through which she had passed and says this gave her "a tremendous feeling of being of use to others apart from my baby." Through working with this post-natal support group, Ella weaned herself from the state of total immersion in her baby. It is this period that can be so long and drawn-out and painful for the so-cially isolated mother.

Feeling Tired

First-time older mothers, unlike those who already have families, often remark on the tiredness, anxiety, and even panic they experience, especially in the early days.

> Both of us were terrified. Having had no contact with infants, we relied on books. I put myself into voluntary purdah, determined not to surface until I had estab-lished my confidence.

Even so, this experience was rewarding because she found the relationship with her husband strengthened by it. "Sharing care of Gemma has been the longest sole period of shared activity in our thirteen years." On the other hand, many of those new mothers who write within two years of a child's birth say that libido is much reduced, they are too exhausted for sex, and make love much less frequently than before conception.

One woman, whose youngest child is now five, says, "The baby was so demanding and I was so tired I am surprised that the marriage survived at all sometimes." She says she had "nothing left over" for her husband, "nothing left to give." The first eighteen months were "a dark, black patch" in her life.

Once this period is over, most couples seem to rediscover their sex lives if they have not grown apart, with diametrically opposed social roles and responsibilities, in the meantime.

At forty-five, with children of twenty, eighteen, fourteen, and ten weeks, Diana is enjoying the changed form of the family, which now spreads across three generations (since her mother is alive); she says that the birth has "thrilled and rejuvenated" her. Diana claims that:

> The adventure of producing and supporting this new personality is more interesting than the alternatives of middle-age-career, more holidays, and outings. Our new arrival has come at an age when many of our friends are tired, bored, frustrated, and wondering what to do with themselves!

Life After the Baby Comes

She and her husband feel the experience has made life richer, and they feel much younger.

It is obvious that it is not just a question of learning new and difficult technical tasks. For the woman who has been until then exclusively career-oriented and engaged in work which has a beginning, middle, and end, caring for a baby for the first time poses an entirely new activity of a kind that is never finished and that she can never assess completely. As one woman put it:

> I find it difficult with young children to work at full stretch with my attention divided in several different directions at once. Having been exhorted at school to "Keep your eye on the ball" and "concentrate on the job at hand," I was not prepared for this.

Another, listing the things she has learned since she had her baby, says they are: 1) rarely finishing a conversation; 2) never eating a meal leisurely; 3) drinking cold tea and coffee; and 4) getting jobs done while the baby is asleep. All this makes her feel that external events are "manipulating" her. This is sometimes made more acute for the woman who has had her first baby in her late thirties because of what one woman calls "a heightened awareness of problems and perhaps taking the whole experience more seriously, as a commitment and responsibility." It is this, rather than simply a failure in resilience or lack of physical energy, which proves most tiring. Many women say they go on in faith, not really knowing whether they are doing well or badly. There are a million and one tasks, repetitive and mundane, none of which are rewarded and most of which go unnoticed by anybody, but these are only incidental to the main activity, which is completely amorphous and which continues day and night. To have to face this alone and without the support of a loving partner can be a nightmare.

Yet having a partner and other family members involved does not necessarily make it any simpler. For though it is possible to draw sustenance from their concern and caring, the birth means that radical changes have to be worked through together and new understanding sought, and this can be a painful process. Tiredness and confusion may mean that communication breaks down, and that the person who is most trying to help proves to be the most irritating. The birth of a child in an already formed family, or to a couple who have been sometime together and have formed a *modus vivendi* for just the two of them, compels adjustment in a whole network of relationships. People caught up in this begin to see themselves and each other in a new light. It can be a major growth experience in middle age.

7

Partners

B abies thrive when they are cared for by more than one loving adult. This simple fact, reflecting the kind of cherishing in the family that babies receive all over the world, has been obscured by psychological pronouncements on the part of experts who have threatened mothers with causing incalculable damage to their infants if they did not commit themselves to full-time mothering, day in and day out, for the first three years of the child's life.

The power of John Bowlby's work[1] to grip women with fear that they were neglecting and depriving their children when they handed them over to another adult for a well-earned break affected a whole generation of mothers, and often made them feel resentful of the baby who was trapping them within four walls, and guilty that they felt the resentment. It was not, of course, Dr. Bowlby's fault. His research was caught up in an insidious social force which in the fifties was driving women back to the homes to be good wives and mothers and telling them that they ought to find all their fulfillment there. If you could not, you were not a "real" woman. Mothers reared children, collected cotton spools and empty cartons to make educational playthings, baked bread, and cultivated the home arts as if their lives depended on it. We thought we were doing the best for our children. Some struggled to do things outside the home as well, but without our husbands or children noticing.

Indoctrinating a mother with the notion that she is the one person who matters in her child's life is one element in the suppression of women as potential wage-earners and creators outside the purely domestic sphere. Domestic work has always been second class.

It is easy for a mother to make herself essential to a small child, easy to build such an intense one-to-one relationship, with no room for any other adult's participation, that the child cannot be left with anyone else, will not accept comfort from them, and suffers an acute trauma of separation if the mother attempts to cut the bond. The woman whose only emotional rewards are in her family may make herself indispensable to her children because otherwise she is nothing.

In societies in which other family members and friends and neighbors share in the care of small children, the child moves easily from one to the other. Of course she knows who her mother is, even if the compound is shared with her co-wives and their children, but the relationship is not so exclusive that it rules out other attachments. The mother-child tie is one of a whole pattern of rich relationships. Among the Ganda, researchers Schaffer and Emerson[2] found that by the time babies were eighteen months old, all but a handful of

128

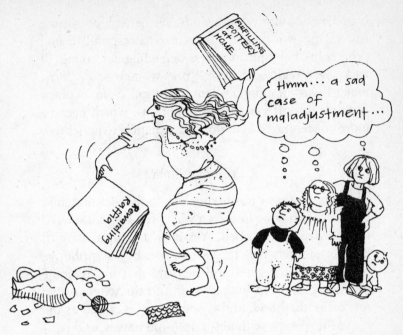

Women ought to find their fulfillment in the home . . .

children were emotionally attached to more than one person, and often to several. The father was most likely to be the chief of these attachment figures. But toddlers were also attached to older children who acted as caregivers.

There is a very special time in the life of any mother and baby when the relationship is intense in a different way, which I touched on earlier. This is during the first six to eight weeks of the child's life, the period that Donald Winnicott called that of "primary maternal preoccupation," when the psychophysiological bond of a lactating mother to her infant is often so strong that it preempts other relationships, seems to blot out the rest of the world, and causes her to respond to and protect her baby like a tigress defending her young. "I had never realized before," one woman said, "how much I was an animal—gloriously so." Some women say that this affects all their emotions, which become more concentrated and more passionately experienced.

A Primitive Bond

This phase of new motherhood is so distinct that any-body else behaving in such a way would be considered pathologically disturbed. Yet it is a natural part of being a mother. It is the recognition of this primitive bond between mother and neonate that has in some ways been allowed to spill over into the whole of the rest of motherhood, and is sometimes accepted as the norm for women with ten-month-old babies, and two-year-old and four-year-old and eight-year-old children. When the mother cannot function in this emotional intensity or feels crushed by the emotional demands made on her psyche, she believes there must be some-thing wrong with her.

The woman starting out on motherhood in her thir-ties or forties for the first time is often rather afraid of this. She has watched other women with babies and from the vantage point of her career has seen what has happened to fellow students and colleagues. This may be one reason why she has put off having a child. She wanted freedom to live her own life first, to put her education to some use, to achieve something. As one put it, "I needed to protect my individuality." Another said, "I feel I was conditioned by what everyone else wanted to do or has done. I needed to free myself to think out what I wanted to do and make it my own decision." And yet another, "I was an independent, ambitious career woman with a happy marriage based on the principle of equality. I regard this stage of motherhood [with little ones] as temporary and a temporary pause in my career development. I imagine I will return to my former dynamic, individual, ambitious self. If I had had a baby in my twenties I would have found motherhood claustrophobic, crippling my independence and freedom. I couldn't even consider marriage then, so strong was my desire to be free."

She is sometimes aware that in a way she "mothers" her partner and is anxious lest the baby's claims for attention compete with his. It is important for them to discuss such anxieties in advance of the birth. A good prenatal class in which there is plenty of free discussion and sharing between expectant parents lets them do just that and discover that other couples have the same doubts and apprehensions. Penny and Leo have been together five years. His mother left him as a baby and he was brought up by his father. Penny said she knew she mothered him: "That side is strong in our relationship. Sometimes he says, 'I won't be your baby anymore' . . . oh! that sounds soppy! He feels threatened by the baby. But I have seen him with small babies and he's lovely with them. I've tried to reassure him."

Prue comments on what Penny is saying: "I feel the same with my husband. It was my decision to have the baby and there was no encouragement. But I've seen him with children. He's changed a lot with the pregnancy. First of all he wasn't interested at all. He was worried and said, 'I don't feel old enough to have a family.' He didn't want to be tied down. Now he's looking forward to it . . . he's totally changed."

Lyn says: "When I first realized I was pregnant, Dick's attitude was, 'Oh God!' He used to treat children like Martians, incomprehensible! He stood back from them. Now I've noticed him seeming more relaxed, not just with children, but a kind of emotional freedom. He used to be very self-contained emotionally. The pregnancy has given a legitimate channel for feelings which have been kept out and which he has never expressed before. This has had a very positive effect on our relationship."

The dynamics of psychological change when a couple share together the emotional as well as the physical preparation for a baby are such that each is better able to meet the stresses that come after and enjoy the inevitable change in their relationship. As one woman said, it was not only that they were very happy about the pregnancy, it was also a "bonding" of two people.

Shared Responsibility

A loving partner who shares parenting with an equal sense of responsibility is the foundation of life for those women who describe themselves as happy and confident mothers. One woman looking back eighteen years later to the birth of her twins at thirty-five and the subsequent experience of parenting with a husband who, she says, "took a full share in caring for the children from the start" comments:

We have discovered ourselves. There is a whole area of one's character that emerges in parenthood, in the way one copes . . . and in communicating with one's children. This has been a continuing surprise over the years.

This partner is often a husband, sometimes a lover, sometimes another woman, but the woman alone without anyone to share parenting, or who struggles to bring up a child while her partner is immersed in career and success outside the home, is invariably at a disadvantage. The majority of women who wrote made explicit statements about ways in which they worked out together their joint commitment as parents. The woman having her first baby at this age who has worked outside the home over a period of some years, together sharing household chores in an egalitarian way, is more likely to plan a strategy of this kind with her partner than women who already have families and who go on to have another baby or start another family after an interval, sometimes with a new husband. It is the middle-aged second husband who tends to see his main responsibilities as outside the home and to leave child care exclusively to his wife.

But for any man who feels under pressure at work and is climbing a career ladder, home tends to be "off-duty" time when peace and quiet, contentment and some conviviality are expected. He feels under heavy financial responsibility and looks on home as a place of relaxation where he can enjoy an interval with his wife and child. These are the fathers who play with their children and sometimes "help" but who feel no responsibility for child care. Some of these women who are left "holding the baby" sound a note of regret and some obviously feel trapped in their roles as mothers, at least for the time being, and are critical of the absent partner.

Olivia had one child at twenty-seven and her second at thirty-six, after being told by her gynecologist that she would not be able to have any more children and failing to adopt. Laurence is a university lecturer. Olivia says that he helped much more with the first baby, because "he was very jealous of my ability to feed him and wanted to do everything for him that he could. This time Laurence isn't at home as much. His job is very demanding and time-consuming and he travels away from home frequently. He has perhaps changed the baby's diaper a dozen times in seventeen months and gets up with her in the morning once a week if I'm lucky. Our roles have become more 'typed' than ten years ago. Laurence's work has very high priority for all of us. We don't have the equality of job prospects that we shared in our early twenties."

Una is forty, with children aged thirteen, eleven, and nine, and before the birth of her new baby was a part-time college lecturer. Her husband has long days in the office and gets home late, so does not help with the domestic work or the children. Una says, "I wonder whether I shall ever be able to get a job now, with my age and the numbers of unemployed increasing together. I have pangs of jealousy at my husband's career success, as I was just as brainy and well qualified as he was once. What really bugs me is that if he wants a regular evening out he can have one. If *I* want a regular

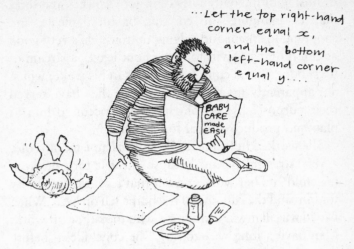

Laurence is a university lecturer . . .

evening out, he says I can have one, but then has to be away with his job." She confesses that she feels intellectually frustrated and resentful.

Teresa has just had her second baby after postpartum depression for a year following her first child's birth. Her firstborn is now two and a quarter, and it is clear from the way she writes that puerperal hormone changes give a very inadequate explanation for the depression into which she is sinking again. Her husband was "thrilled" with the pregnancy but, she says, "I'd have appreciated help with shopping and heavy housework. I deeply resented him for not offering, after I'd said a couple of times I needed help, and I was too proud to go on asking. He thinks of fatherhood as having a 'nice cuddle' and playing with 'pretty, well-cared-for kids,' but should also have the experience of disposing of the daily piles of grubby clothes and dirty diapers, planning and cooking balanced meals, and shopping for them and tidying up toys. He's very good at entertaining David for hours but leaves a stream of toys, books, used cups, and clothes in his wake, which are apparently invisible to him once they have served their purpose. If I go out it doesn't occur to him to plan and produce a meal for the child."

She worked full-time till David was nine months old, a very stressful period because she felt torn between the child and her work and felt that total responsibility for him and the running of the home fell on her. "When David was ill it was always me who took time off work. Men have a long way to go," she concludes, "before they are truly fathers the way women are mothers to their children."

Conditioned Mothers

It is not just that men take it for granted that women are responsible for baby care and domestic work and expect them to be better at looking after babies than they are; it is also that women themselves are socially conditioned to feel *they* ought to be homemakers and child-rearers to such an extent that they may shut the father out of full participation in parenting. Jill, aged thirty-six and doing part-time teaching, cannot help herself, the emotions are so strong. She feels depressed, tired, and "in a state of confusion about my roles of mother/wife/worker," and weighed down by "a terrible responsibility." Yet "even though I trust my husband when he is dealing with Sean, I feel that *I* am on duty.

I hover and remind him of things. He would rather be left to get on with it! Our relationship as a couple has been very much affected. I have become aware that at times I exclude Mike in my baby-centered world . . . we are like ships passing in a fog."

The marriages of some of the mothers who wrote had already broken up under this kind of strain. Hannah, for instance, says that the relationship "foundered under the stress of responsibilities which I was left to bear." They now live on different levels of a big house. She brings up her son, but his father is "his best play-partner and brings him many things which I cannot offer."

The social isolation that many mothers feel with their small children is peculiar to our Western, urban society. In Muslim societies, which represent for many in the West the epitome of female subjugation, women have a vigorous and highly colorful autonomous world in their own quarters, from which men are excluded.[3] A sisterhood of women share in child care, both in the practical tasks and the emotional support of the new mother.

The Indian woman is similarly part of a group consisting of her husband's brothers' wives, his mother, and his unmarried sisters. There is no privacy, but at the same time there is no loneliness.[4]

In the Caribbean women are part of a sisterhood network, helping, gossiping about, counseling, and sharing with each other, bemoaning their lot at the hands of men who are good for nothing, and striving in common to feed their children, clothe them, get them through school, and "grow them right." In each village

three leaders, all women, act as primary communica-
tors between every household: the postmistress, the
schoolmistress, and the midwife.[5] In rural areas, to be
isolated is impossible, and the same pattern of social
organization infiltrates the life of the clusters of shack
dwellings and the homes of the poor in the towns.

Women are often told that depression suffered after
childbirth is the result of major hormonal changes and
the distress they feel is all put down to physiological
processes over which they have no control. Though
this may be cheering for some, for at least it is not their
"fault," it perpetuates the misery for many women,
who are thereby absolved from the responsibility or
opportunity to change the social conditions in which
they function from day to day as mothers, which are
the real cause of their distress. It is only too easy for
a man, too, to explain his wife's depression by reference
to her hormones and, apart from urging her to see the
doctor, do nothing else about it. If she does go to the
doctor, drug treatment often does not cure her. A controlled trial of the commonly prescribed antidepressant
imipramine revealed that it was no better than a pla-
cebo.[6]

To be alone in a house with total responsibility for
a screaming baby who seems to be crying *at* you and
telling you what a hopeless mother you are is a *social*
situation which has nothing to do with whether you
have a uterus and breasts. One woman said, "I go and
hide in the bathroom when she cries. Maybe I do that
instead of flinging her down the stairwell." It is not
only mothers who do this. Distraught babysitters who
cannot quiet the infant do it too.

138

Physicians, public health nurses, health visitors, childbirth educators, and other counselors continue to reassure the new mother that all that is needed is a readjustment of hormones, an attitude that stems from a uterine psychology that had its origins in the Middle Ages and from concepts of hysteria as the result of a wandering womb. Freudian theory reinforced this ideology of the female mind as a direct consequence of anatomy and laid down that a woman's reproductive system was "the site for the acting out of impulses, especially aggression, and its derivative, sex anxiety, and maternity-pregnancy fears."[7] No such claims have been made about men's mood swings, the inference being that they are more purely cerebral and less chained to their physiology. Yet, as Ann Oakley points out,[8] monthly cycles have been reported for men in body temperature,[9] weight,[10] and beard growth,[11] and pain threshold and cyclical rhythms have been discovered in emotional changes,[12] urine levels of hormones,[13] and schizophrenia, manic depression, and epilepsy.[14]

The Father's Role

In fact it cannot be assumed that women are the only ones to experience postpartum depression. Childbirth is a major life crisis for many couples, and becoming a father can be just as stressful for a man as the transition to motherhood is for a woman. Sometimes a man is so overwhelmed by his own feelings that he is unable to give the woman the emotional support she needs. As men get more involved in the experience of birth, not just as watchers or members of a supporting cast, but as full emotional participants, they encounter many of the psychological conflicts that are typical of the passage to new social roles. They, too, experience the primary preoccupation with the baby, which until now has been thought to be a female characteristic.

If it is believed that men must always be strong, that they must not show their emotions, and that their main task is to provide economic support, leaving all the feeling to the woman, this may be seen as an unfortunate social development. But in fact this emotional involvement means that couples have a chance to share in being parents and be open with each other as never before. Those who experience it find it an enriching and often completely unexpected bonus of parenthood.

It can be hard for a man to get involved with a baby and bond with it when it has been produced by the hospital as a specialist medical product and he feels that the whole process of having a baby is so risky that it is best to leave it all to the "experts." Fathers, like mothers, also find it difficult to develop confidence in handling the baby if they feel they are second-rate caregivers and that someone is watching to see that they do it properly. There are some situations in which both parents are more likely to feel that the baby is the property of the hospital and to be very apprehensive about taking on responsibility for this precious new life. When a baby has been in intensive care, especially in a hospital where parent participation is not encouraged, a man may feel so anxious that the simplest solution seems to him to be to get out of the house and concentrate on his work.

In those intensive care nurseries, however, where

both parents are welcome at any time of the day or night and are shown how they can help look after their baby, confidence develops very early on. Most of the studies that have been published about this emphasize the benefits for the mother.[15] But the effect on the father is often astonishing, and changes an understandable hesitation and fear in handling his baby to supercompetence and pleasure in a matter of a few hours. The self-confidence he develops then indirectly can help the mother, too, and gives her the emotional support she needs. It sometimes seems that the emotional energy that is released when a man tends to his very tiny or sick baby flows beyond the infant and in a mysterious way enables the mother to feel cherished, too. Perhaps not having to go on as if nothing has happened and keep a stiff upper lip allows him to come closer to her feelings so that they share this difficult emotional journey with more understanding of each other's vulnerability.

Though Michael's first view of his eight-week premature twins in intensive care was, he says, "very fearsome" because they were wired up to "things going bleep, bleep, bop," he says that when he visited the unit after that first time he hardly noticed the apparatus, only his babies. He had to overcome apprehension about interfering with the smooth running of the unit, but quickly realized that the staff were welcoming and wanted him there: "We were all in it together."

One of the babies was suffering from RDS, respiratory distress syndrome, because her lungs were inadequately inflated. Their normal lining, like the bubbles in detergent, was only partially present, and as a result her lungs collapsed between each breath and the sides stuck together like plastic bags. Then she had to make a terrific gasping effort to take the next breath.

Michael stood over her in the plastic box in which she struggled for life, feeling helpless to do anything, until a nurse suggested that he should hold her hand. As he did so he felt not only compassion and love, but as if the baby were giving *him* comfort. He started to stroke the little arm and talk to her soothingly. "She seemed to relax," he said. The baby was linked to an apparatus that measured the amount of oxygen in her blood. He had been shown how to read this, and to his surprise he saw that when he stimulated her in this way the oxygen content went up from about sixty to ninety. After three-quarters of an hour doing this he noticed that she liked the inside of her thigh stroked and seemed to "feel safer." She began to breathe more easily, and he again saw the results on the oxygen meter.

Michael's relationship with his baby is a far cry from that of another father, who though, his wife Janet says, he is "close" to his son, needed her encouragement to "become involved on the physical side, changing diapers, bathing him, feeding him, etc. As with most domestic matters," she explains, "he'd rather not be involved so, and finds it easier now the child is two and a half, can communicate, and is not just an object with needs." This baby was born six weeks early by cesarean section and spent time in an intensive care unit that was less liberal and welcoming to parents. He developed jaundice and was taken back there again. Though she does not say how her husband feels, Janet says she felt "intimidated" while in the hospital.

Partners

Breaking Down Barriers

A father's relationship with his new baby affects his relationship with his wife, too. It may have been partly because Michael was so stirred by the experience with his little daughter that he could be honest about his emotions with his wife. She said, "I can have a good cry without him thinking I'm stupid, and if he weeps I don't think, 'You're a man. You're not supposed to cry.' " They were able to support each other in a way that is impossible if a couple relies on artificial hope and cheerfulness all the time. This partnership continued after the babies were home and is a firm basis from which they cope with the household disruption and sheer hard work that twins inevitably entail.

But it is not, of course, only when things are difficult that a partner is needed. Many women write of the joy they experience when childbirth is shared, and say, "I could not have done it without him there." Many say that the man's presence during labor and his emotional surrender at delivery is profoundly moving for them and that they will never forget this time. For the newly delivered woman it is not only the sight and feeling of the newborn lying on her body that is deeply moving, but what this means to her partner and his spontaneous emotional release into tears, laughter, and caresses. One man just said very slowly and clearly, "Wow . . . wooow . . . wooooow!" Not all fathers express themselves with dramatic abandon! Another, after having kissed his wife and told her how clever she was, picked up the baby and danced around the room with her, singing "Waltzing Matilda." Some women say that although they did not have any strong sense that the baby belonged to them following delivery, when they saw the baby held in its father's arms and *his* response to his child, there was a rush of emotion and they promptly fell in love.

Sara and Philip decided to have their second baby at home. Philip describes it:

> It is hard, impossible, to communicate to others the joy and wonder I experienced as my son slid out of Sara and with his mother's help onto her breast. Dan's tongue was belting away as if he had crawled into a desert oasis and was searching for the life-sustaining nectar.

Sara handed the baby to Philip as she delivered the placenta. "For the first time the reality of this life creation that Sara and I had shared for nine months was driven home . . . The birth of one's own child is," he says, "the happiest, most powerful experience a man can hope to witness." When the midwife had gone home they slept the rest of the night with their little daughter, too, all four together in the large bed. "She was curled against me," said Sara, "and Dan with Philip."

It seems that the intensity of such an experience for both parents prepares the way for powerful emotions which follow. Many couples say, "We are closer." One woman added, "In labor I learned to trust him absolutely. When Jake was born we were so deeply moved. Somehow that deepened our understanding of each other."

The birth is only one point in an emotional journey

together that involves transformations in a couple's relationship as the child grows and as they discover new aspects of themselves. Sometimes these discoveries can be disconcerting, and the changes invariably produce fresh stresses as well as a new closeness, sharpening and further defining the elements of their partnership. One man, asked by his wife how he felt the birth of their daughter, now two years old, had affected their relationship, said, "It's strengthened the pluses of our marriage and deepened the minuses."

Birth need not be an isolated emotional "trip," though it is often reduced to that. It is part of a continuum in the relationship. Sharing in the birth of the child is a psychological experience of such significance that it gives an opportunity for two people to go on from there to evolve a richer life together as caring, sharing parents as well as lovers.

8

Coping
with the Family

"We found it surprisingly hard to tell the other children we were expecting the baby," Roberta says. "We finished up by being rather mysterious, which we hadn't intended, so they started making guesses along the lines of 'Are we getting a color TV?'"

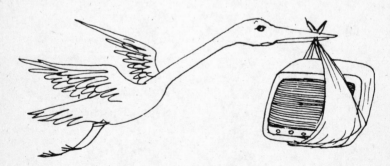

Are we getting a color TV?

Coping with the Family

Ann, too, writes:

> I found it awkward to tell the children. Eventually, at
> about four and a half months, after getting them to-
> gether one Saturday morning, Simon asked them to
> guess our news. They guessed we were divorcing, sep-
> arating, going abroad, that he'd been fired, but none
> guessed correctly. They were amazed. The boys (twenty
> and eighteen) were easygoing and thought it was "a
> good idea," but Susan (fourteen) left the room and
> became very quiet. The next day she implied that it
> was thoughtless of us to let this happen. . . .

Couples having a second family after a gap find the
most difficult people to tell are their adolescent children. It is almost as if the open acknowledgment of
sexual activity between parents compromises the young
people in their own sexual identity. Boys away at school
may be horrified, and at this age they tend to be embarrassed by having a mother who looks pregnant.
Girls say, "How *could* you, Mother!" as if she were
discovered in some gross impropriety. One girl said to
her father, "You *naughty* boy, Daddy!" and he was
embarrassed in his turn. A boy of eleven exclaimed,
"Oh, Mom, now you've gone and done it!" and a little
later, "I hope it drowns!" He would not touch his
mother right through pregnancy or, at first, the baby.
Another seemed concerned about his mother, but only,
she suggests, because he wanted to be sure she could
continue to cook his dinner!

Ingrid says of her fourteen-year-old, "She worried
about her friends' reactions to my appearance and her
studies being impaired by 'a screaming baby.'" An-

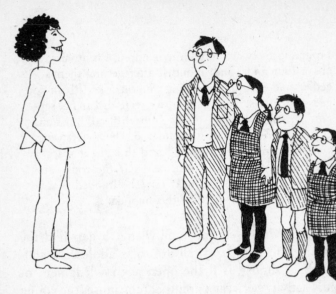

I found it awkward to tell the children

other girl of this age "went through two very traumatic years and definitely resented the intrusion of noise, demands, toys, and diapers, and the time consumed by a baby. Whether her adolescent years would have been so difficult without the child, I don't know, but in suffering we grow as people and at nearly seventeen she has become well balanced," her mother says.

Loneliness

Older boys who have already gained some confidence in their own identity seem to cope well with the experience, while girls under about the age of fourteen may identify with their mother in a very caring and

148

compassionate way and sometimes worry for her. One woman says that her daughter of twelve bought diapers out of her pocket money. Frances, a single mother with a daughter of ten who has just had another baby, says she did not realize how lonely her daughter had been:

> She was fantastically excited and got involved in my childbirth class—counting herself my partner, reading all the books. She was very good with the relaxation exercises. She cried when I lit a cigarette or had a drink, so I stopped. She was all the things supportive partners are supposed to be. Toward the end of the pregnancy she got very tense. We must have had the largest list of phone numbers and emergency procedures!

Anna feels that her pregnancy is a very good experience for her daughter of thirteen and says she has "shared" it:

> I have tried to keep her in touch with all my body changes and she has seen me naked. I feel it will be a help to her in the future to have absorbed all this, rather than come to it "cold" as I did.

However the information is received initially, most families seem to adjust not only well but with delight to a late addition. The boy who would not touch his mother or the baby started playing with his sister in her first year, though roughly ("she loved it," his mother said), and is now "very tender and attached." Women say that it brings out a newfound tenderness in their sons and believe that it is a very positive preparation for later fatherhood. The "macho" typical of many male adolescents' picture of themselves gives way to gentleness and concern, and the whole family benefits. They no longer tear through the house with gangs of youths, and even the stereos may be turned down. "Our family life has become softer and more caring," one woman says. A sixteen-year-old big brother changes his baby sister's diapers and is very gentle and playful with her. "He's mind-blowing," an eighteen-year-old says of his newborn brother; "terrific," a sixteen-year-old of a baby sister. An older brother of twenty remarks that he likes the changed form of the family now that it cuts right across the generations and, he feels, unites them all.

After she has adjusted to the idea, an adolescent daughter may become much closer to her mother in a shared womanhood, sometimes even in a kind of female conspiracy against men. One mother said of her daughter:

> She became more and more involved and helpful. She offered to stay with me for the birth, to be "a reliable help, unlike Daddy" as she put it.

It may be important for a girl to have time with her mother alone after the birth to discuss her often very conflicting feelings. While mother and baby are in the hospital this is often impossible, and after their return home there are so many visitors and such a lot of work that this time for quiet sharing can be crowded out. Elizabeth says her daughter developed a bad sore throat. They had a "good gossip" together the first time they were alone after the birth. Elly, who had been very excited about the baby coming and involved in all the details of the pregnancy, told her mother that she was worried that she did not love the baby immediately. Elizabeth said *she* felt just like that, too, and that it often took some time to get to know a baby.

Adolescents are good babysitters, though women say that they try not to make this a bind or take it for granted that the older children will give their time; many make a regular arrangement for paying for time spent on this. A mother may find her son mending his motor bike with the baby bouncing in her seat watching the fascinating proceedings. The younger child seems to benefit greatly from all this, though one mother says she is anxious lest the baby, present "during the usual teenage arguments," grows up undisciplined.

Being with older children provides an intellectual stimulus for the baby, but mothers describe ways in which they make sure that the younger child is able to meet children of about the same age, too. They notice how they themselves are enriched by contact with younger women and their children, opening a whole new social world which in the past they might not have thought they would enjoy, but which keeps them in touch with attitudes and concerns of couples still in their twenties.

Listening to Heartbeats

Children between four or five and early adolescence are rarely surprised by a pregnancy, and some have been urging their mothers to have a baby for years. For girls, friends at school who have younger babies at home to look after are considered very special. The changes of pregnancy are followed with curiosity, and women say that this is a great educational opportunity for their older children. Both boys and girls can listen to the baby's heartbeats through a fetal stethoscope. If you know how your baby is lying you may be able to locate the fetal heart yourself without difficulty in the last two or three months of pregnancy.

Lie back against pillows on a couch or bed and first feel with your hands where the most actively moving small knobs are placed at the moment. These are probably the feet and will often be at one side or the other right under your ribs. If the baby is active at the time, an older child can feel the kicks. Follow the legs around to the other side and you will reach the trunk; move down from there, about two hands' breadth, sliding your hand in a little as you do, and you reach the spot where it is probably easiest to hear the fetal heart. You will be at the level of your own umbilicus or below. If the baby has engaged in your pelvis with its head down like an egg in an eggcup, this spot will be below your umbilicus but out to the left or right side. Instead of a stethoscope you can use the cardboard cylinder from the middle of a toilet paper roll or a tumbler with the open end placed over the area where you hope to pick up sounds. When a baby is lying with its back against its mother's spine, the limbs are at the front of your abdomen, and it may be more difficult to detect the heartbeat because the limbs are in front of the chest. If your umbilicus sinks in with a saucer-shaped depression in this area, this is probably the position your baby is in at the moment. If your umbilicus sticks out with a rounded shape like a watermelon behind it, your baby is probably lying in the more usual anterior position and you will find it easier to pick up the heart. In the seventh and eighth months babies change position frequently, often many times a day, so trying another time, when you feel the baby has shifted, may lead to success.

Women described the wonder their older children express when they hear the baby's heartbeats or are helped to locate the different parts of the baby and feel the movements. Prenatal visits are held during school hours, but some mothers take an older child along during her vacation so that she can understand what is happening and indirectly learn more about changes that may well take place in her own body, too, in later years.

Some women having babies when over thirty choose to give birth at home partly because they feel that understanding about and sharing in birth can be important for the other children. The younger the other children, the more the mother is concerned about separation from them; the older they are, the more she sees the birth as a maturational experience for her sons and daughters.

Mary is forty and the older children are aged thirteen, eleven, and nine, a girl and two boys. She says she found that after having amniocentesis she got "hooked into the hospital system" regardless, but was unhappy about the conveyor belt atmosphere of the prenatal clinic and discovered that visiting by other siblings on postnatal wards was on weekends only. So she canceled her appointment and arranged a home birth, a really family-centered experience. When she was in the first stage of labor, "my eldest son came in and was a classic case of pacing up and down, saying, 'Are you all right?' The midwife chatted with him and he became much more relaxed." After the birth her daughter spent several hours just holding the baby. "She called her several times a 'dear little puppy,' and I remembered that a puppy was the only pet she'd had. The feelings about the two must have been similar."

Changing Relationships

When the baby is born new patterns of relationships in the family emerge. If a woman is preoccupied with her baby or feeling tired, older children tend to turn to their father more and also to become more self-reliant. This is very different from the more usual change in pattern when a newborn is introduced into a family where the older children are still under about five years. There an older child, the displaced baby, may regress temporarily. A typical description of the mother of a two-year-old after the birth of a new baby is:

> When Dinah came to visit me she had a good look at the baby and then got very fussy and noisy. My husband was suffering from a hangover so each bang and clatter made him wince. When we came home she would poke him through the bars of his cot "to see if he's awake." The poor child suffered from lack of sleep for a few weeks. When I was feeding Joe she would say she wanted a wee, so I would either have to have the potty chair in the room with me or try to get Dinah

on the toilet with Joe hanging on to his means of nour-
ishment for grim life.

With older children the mother often has the opposite impression: they grow up. She starts to see them
through new eyes and is often astonished at the blos-
soming of qualities of caring and tenderness that she
did not realize they possessed. One woman, commenting on the relationship of her three teenagers with
their baby brother, says: "They have all been so positive
and beautiful with him that this must be one of the
biggest pluses of all." And a father, summing up the
effect of the birth on the older children, aged twenty
down to fourteen, says: "All seem to enjoy the change
in structure that the baby has brought. Each child feels
much more mature and responsible. . . . It has given
the family a focus."

One disadvantage of having a baby later on, however, is that grandparents are not always alive, or well
enough, to share in the joy of the new baby. Mothers
see this as a sadness for them and a loss for the child.
Some women feel torn between wanting to care for a
sick parent and the child's needs as he or she grows
and finds it a great strain. Several women, however,
described how a grandmother who was ill, or who had
lost interest in life, gained a new sparkle with the birth
of the baby. Some of these grandmothers had recently
lost their husbands and were obviously still grieving
painfully. The arrival of a baby helped them to come
out of a sometimes prolonged mourning and had enormous psychological benefits for them.

A woman most appreciates a mother who lives near

enough to offer regular practical help, rather than advice. As one says: "She has the baby for an hour at a time and allows me to recharge my batteries." It is sometimes possible to make friends with an older person in the neighborhood you can trust who can learn your ways and take over occasionally. An adopted grandmother or father provides a child with another loving adult, and the relationship brings great pleasure to an otherwise lonely older person.

Some grandmothers see the baby as a threat to them, depriving them of love they need from their son or daughter. The new mother then feels an extra drain on her strength as she tries to cope with the emotional demands of a lonely and unhappy parent as well as stresses of dealing with a family, new baby, and running a home. She may become very resentful of this parent, whether it is her own or her partner's mother, and it is important that the couple discuss their feelings together and develop a joint strategy to cope with the problem.

The birth of a child can profoundly affect the relationship of a woman with her own mother. This change may start in pregnancy. One woman, four months pregnant, says: "My parents have, at last, realized that I'm 'grown up' now and think twice before telling me what to do." Some women remain in an almost adolescent relation with their mothers until they have their first baby. If this is not till they are after thirty, the bond between mother and daughter has become hard-set, the older woman treating her daughter as irresponsible, incompetent, and in need of protection, and the younger in a continual state of revolt.

Coping with the Family

Mothers

Part of the sense of freedom and of having matured which some women over thirty experience when they have a baby is that this relationship with their own mother undergoes rapid change. However concerned the older woman is that her daughter cannot look after a baby properly, and even if she offers unwelcome advice in the first few months, after a while she usually begins to realize that she *can*. One woman said that recovering the happy relationship with her own mother, which she feels came with surrendering her defensiveness and learning to give love, brought deep satisfaction. "I am sure I was arrogant and selfish before. Loving a little baby is the completest joy."

Where a woman already has a good relationship with her mother, the sharing between the two women further enriches it. Di said the fact that her mother had successfully breastfed four of them helped develop her own confidence in breastfeeding. Her mother came to stay for a few weeks:

> We've always been close, but for the first time I really understood the mother/child relationship. She never criticized anything I did, was interested in new ways of doing things, and was able to take my outbursts of temper (mainly due to tiredness) completely in her stride. She was my safety valve.

Where sisters are emotionally close and noncompetitive the new mother may find they can give her very good postnatal support. It is best not to have to get to know new people when you are most in need of an understanding friend to listen and give relaxed counseling and not be judgmental. Connie, whose two sisters gave her a great deal of support over the telephone, added that she also had a marvelous cleaning lady and a freezer full of cooked foods; these practical aspects of life can loom large after a baby comes. Some women, though they have sisters who have had babies, cannot happily use them to help during this period because they are still competing with them. Sometimes one element in actually having the baby is that a woman is locked in competition with a sister and wants to prove to her mother or father than she can do as well as her sister.

For most women a mother-in-law, even a very understanding one, is classed as a "visitor" as compared with one's own mother. On the other hand, the birth of the baby may bring the new mother and her mother-in-law closer together. A woman of thirty-six says: "Since the birth, my relationship with my mother-in-law has improved enormously. I did not feel any particular affinity with her for a long time, and she herself was probably thinking that I might not be good enough for HER SON! When she saw how well I was coping with the pregnancy, she already considered me better, but it was really on the day of the birth that the sudden change occurred. She was delighted with the baby, and in fact I think she was proud of me as well, as I did so well with the birth. And as her son thanked her for her giving birth to him as a baby ('Now I realize what *you* did!') she really blossomed into an even brighter smile, and her eyes were shining with the joy of being recognized, maybe for the first time in her life, and that by her son!"

Sometimes a new mother knows already that she cannot cope with her mother-in-law for more than short periods at a time and that these have to be carefully planned in advance. If this is so, it is vital to discuss it with your husband so that he knows the strategy, realizes that you need his protection at this stage, and is not left feeling disloyal to both women. Connie, who got on so well with her own mother, was usually great friends with her husband's mother, too. But the two women could not agree about Connie's style of breast-feeding, and she knew that her mother-in-law was worried about prolonged breastfeeding and Dan getting interrupted sleep at nights. The baby was breastfed whenever she wanted until she was sixteen months. At fifteen months she had a throat infection and rejected other foods, having fourteen feeds a day, not including the night ones. "I know," said Connie, "because my mother-in-law, whom we were staying with and who was disgusted with the whole thing, had counted for me!" Once the infection cleared up, however, she weaned herself in four days. "That was one up on my mother-in-law, who is actually normally a very understanding person."

This is one of the bonuses of breastfeeding, that it is the perfect food if the child is ill and may be not only the most comforting one, but also the only one that the child can digest and wants. In my own experience most of the crises in breastfeeding, when women seek help urgently, together with anxiety about not yet having weaned a child, come at times of the year when there are family gatherings and when members of the family go to stay with each other, such as Christmas and Easter or the summer holidays.

In some ways the older mother is immunized from the criticisms of those to whom she is nearest by her own experience of life. She knows that there is more than one way of doing things and that they probably all work. She is, as one woman put it, "less of a perfectionist and more of a human being," and is better able to relax and enjoy her baby than she would have been in her twenties.

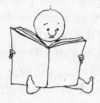

9

Coping Alone

The woman alone faces special challenges in pregnancy, if only because she feels the whole burden of responsibility for planning ahead, for supporting the child financially, for loving it, rests on her shoulders. A woman over thirty tends to take this on with understanding born from her experience of life, probably much more than someone still in her teens or twenties would have.

For some women deciding to have a baby when they are in their thirties, the child is their "last chance" and conception is the consequence of a carefully thought-out decision that this is what they want. Some cannot find the right man with which to form a partnership and are concerned only to have a child. Some do not wish to have a man anyway and prefer a loving relationship with another woman. The lesbian mother is usually not alone, and the relationship with her partner is often a good deal more stable than many heterosexual relationships. The woman who chooses artificial insemination has also taken time to work out what she wants, and the conception is far from the accident that it often is in a male-female partnership.

Other women are having a child after a separation from the baby's father and occasionally after his death. The woman alone is, therefore, not one person but many, who may in fact have little in common.

The woman who has no partner needs a good support network both before and after the baby comes. To start with, it is vital that she has a labor companion who goes with her to childbirth classes, works with her on breathing and relaxation, and understands exactly how to help in labor. To plan on having someone at the birth simply to hold your hand is not enough. You need someone really to share the labor and who has the skills to help you keep on an even course. This can be a woman friend, sister or other relative, childbirth educator or someone studying to be one, and I have known women who have had a trusted man friend take this on, too. A charming and sophisticated older man attended every single childbirth class in a course, on time even when his friend was late, accepting the responsibility because the father of her child was in his late teens and could not face it. He was present throughout the labor and delivery, experienced the rush of emotions that a new father usually does, and then had to stand back as the younger man decided that he liked the idea of being a father after all now that the baby was safely born.

Coping Alone

Labor Companions

Another woman selected two of her lovers as labor companions. They were, according to the midwife, both "marvelous," and, she added, "I'm not sure which I would have chosen!" Another woman spent the major part of the first stage of labor with friends who lived near the hospital, a couple whom she had gotten to know in the prenatal class and whose baby was three weeks old. The father of this other baby had support techniques fresh in his mind, and had learned from his wife's experience, so he shepherded her through to eight centimeters dilation with masterly skill.

The important thing is that the single woman has someone with her whose task it is to concentrate on her needs as a person, not a reproductive body, and whose responsibilities should not be divided between this relationship and medical tasks. This is why it is not enough to rely on a midwife for this, however kind and caring she is.

Still in some hospitals a woman may be left alone in labor. Still when labor wards are full, drugs may be used by busy staff members in place of personal help and understanding. Pat says she went into the hospital far too early, probably because she was alone and felt she would not be able to cope by herself if she left it until contractions were coming five minutes apart:

The contractions stopped for about twelve hours, but it was nice because they weren't busy and the nurses all talked about how I was going to manage on my own and seemed genuinely interested. Unfortunately,

163

Andrew decided to be born at their busy time, and the entirely unsympathetic night staff had taken over. I was totally out of control, couldn't do any of the exercises I'd practiced so assiduously and felt like a complete coward. In the end, they gave me an injection and put me out.

An alternative arrangement is for this companion to be with you at home so that you can spend early labor in familiar surroundings, rather than only to turn up at the hospital. It helps to get into the rhythm of breathing and relaxing in the first half of the first stage in a close partnership, without the intrusion of other people if this can be avoided. Susan, whose lover was abroad and whom she did not want to involve any more than he wished, because she had not consulted him about starting the pregnancy, says that no one can ever talk to her of independence who has not made the journey alone to a hospital to have a baby, and then, three days later, come out of it, going down to the parking lot, collecting the baby at the maternity entrance, and driving off.

A labor companion should have the knowledge to be able to be a "patient advocate," if necessary. A woman in labor needs to be able to rely on someone to say if she is in the middle of a contraction and does not wish to have an injection of Demerol, to remind her that she should be given a vaginal examination immediately before having an epidural just in case she is already almost fully dilated, perhaps to say, before an episiotomy (a surgical cut to enlarge the birth opening) is done, that her friend did hope she might be able to manage without one and would it be possible to see if "breathing the baby out" would help. A patient advocate cannot, by definition, be an employee of the hospital. Anybody working for the hospital is bound to have divided loyalties. To say this may be hurtful to a nurse who sees her role as being on her patient's side, but as Norma Swenson[1] of the Boston Women's Health Collective points out, though attractive as a concept, an alliance between consumers and professionals is unrealistic because the woman having a baby has transient and unequal status in the hospital system.

Sometimes a labor companion can attend at least some of the prenatal visits, too, and look around the maternity unit in advance. Someone unfamiliar with hospitals may find this especially helpful. One woman, reluctant about getting fully involved with her partner's birth, felt much more relaxed about this after meeting hospital staff and finding them friendly. She said she now began to see her role more clearly and would not feel out of place.

Powerful Emotions

With other partners, just as with husbands, powerful emotions are often involved, and it is a mistake to think that a labor companion is there simply to remind you of exercises or rub your back. I remember one man, married with two small children, who had been present at the births of both of them, who supported his mistress through a pregnancy with his child, doing so because he felt it was right, but unwilling to break up his marriage. Duty, responsibility, compassion, whatever he felt, gave way to a passionate outpouring of emotion as he relived the births of his other children. He expressed his pain and joy, and in some inexplicable way this assurance of his emotional surrender to the experience gave the woman who was bearing his child great psychological support.

Another, attending classes with her lesbian partner, had herself had a pregnancy the previous year which had finished in a late miscarriage. It must have been stressful for her to allow herself to identify completely with the woman having the baby and give herself completely to her in loving support, but she did so.

Sometimes the choice of support partner is a woman's own mother. It is vitally important for the mother to share preparation with her daughter if she is to be with her in labor. Not only have birth styles changed, with apparatus in the labor room that the mother may not have seen before, but women tend to bring their own experiences of childbearing with them into the birth they attend. If these were unhappy the mother may not be able to help her daughter gain confidence.

Faith's mother was deeply distressed to learn that her daughter was pregnant. She prayed that she be saved from sin every day. She did not know what to do, whether to turn Faith away or look forward to the birth of the baby with her. She spoke to the pastor at the evangelical church she attended who suggested that the right thing was to give her daughter her unconditional love. Faith was very happy with her mother's changed attitude, and at my suggestion asked her if she would come to childbirth classes with her. She said that her mother had always been very inhibited about anything to do with sex and she did not know how her mother would take all the talk about bodies and feelings. Her labor had been a terrible and frightening ordeal. She had never had another baby because of what she had suffered with Faith. In any event, Faith need not have worried. Her mother, brought up in ignorance of her body, was hungry for information and obviously enjoyed the group, asked questions, discussed vigorously with the other couples present, and told me that her life would have been so different if she had known all this before and had been able to see it for the miracle it was. She supported her daughter magnificently through a drug-free labor, and the two became friends as never before.

The role of the support person can, perhaps, best be illustrated by describing the way a particular partnership worked during a painful induced labor in which a cesarean section was always in the cards and a forceps delivery very likely. The support that this single mother had from another woman during labor gave her the confidence, courage, and trust in her body which resulted in a spontaneous delivery.

Felicia had been warned that she would probably need a cesarean section. She was having a big baby and was of small build. Jo, her friend, had a baby daughter herself. She came to childbirth classes with Felicia, determined to give her full support through what was an emotionally difficult time, not only because of the uncertainty about the birth, but because Felicia was beginning to realize that the father of her baby was not going to leave his wife and children and was very anxious that it might leak out that he had fathered a baby outside the marriage. Both women kept careful notes during as much of the labor as they could and recorded the rest immediately afterward.

Jo's Diary

Jo's diary starts when the midwife rang from the hospital to say that the induction had started and Felicia was asking for her:

> Packed ice into thermos and shot off in taxi. Did relaxing exercises myself in taxi so would bring a calm, reassuring atmosphere with me.

Once there, the first thing she had to do was to work out the best place to stand in the labor room, which was equipped spaceship-style. She needed to be out of the midwife's way, not obstructing the equipment, yet close enough to Felicia to touch and hold her when she seemed to want this. She could see from the clock that each contraction was lasting about forty-five seconds.

> but I felt that the best thing for me to do was to watch Felicia and try to see what she wanted. I didn't watch the time . . . I talked to her between contractions, making her laugh a bit because I felt that was what she needed, and keeping silent with just my hand on her arm during contractions, watching her face and hands and feet to see if they were tensing up, and occasionally just lightly stroking her shoulder for reassurance and to check that it was relaxed. In between contractions I checked that the thermos with ice was nearby and washcloths and lip salve.
>
> I made a point of asking everyone who came in for any length of time what their name was, as I felt that

the more personal the process was, the more confident Felicia would be, and once somebody has given you their name there is less tendency to be high-handed.

After about one and a half hours the contractions were stronger,

> and from now on I didn't move away from her at all. . . . If I moved from one side to let the nurses get at the equipment I moved to the other or held her feet very gently until I could put my hand on her upper arm, which was where she seemed to prefer it.
>
> The machine monitoring the contractions and the baby's heartbeat was not functioning too well, so there was quite a lot of coming and going and tinkering about, which Felicia found distracting. So every time it happened, I told her quietly not to take any notice of them, they weren't important (which must have gone over well with the staff if they heard).

Somebody came to deal with the monitor whom Jo asked firmly but politely to keep his voice down:

> He seemed surprised and obviously thought it rather funny. Then a staff nurse told Felicia to turn over and started to move her mid-contraction. I said quietly, so as not to disturb Felicia, "Could you wait until this contraction is over?" She said, "But she has to turn on her side." I said, "Yes, but not now. Could it wait a minute? Then she could help you herself." It must have carried force because although she looked daggers at me, she waited until I said, "OK," and then we got Felicia over and tried to make her as comfy as possible.

After another two and a quarter hours Felicia said she could not bear any more and she would like some Demerol, but as soon as she had had the injection she started to feel desperate and said she wanted an epidural:

> I told her the Demerol took a quarter of an hour to work, that although it must seem like forever, did she want to try and ride out the quarter hour? I promised I would tell her when it was up. I said that if she didn't want to wait I'd get someone to do the epidural. She said she would wait and between contractions I told her the time and how much longer there was to go till the end of the quarter hour. I could see the Demerol had started to work and I told her and when she said that she was OK told her how well she was doing and how wonderfully she had got through that quarter hour.

Felicia says: "I coped only with Jo. Without her I might have gone under." This is how she describes the help Jo gave her:

> She was encouraging me all the time, saying "relax into it—you're doing very well—very good," and praising and encouraging me. Throughout, a battery of doctors and nurses kept coming in, and the monitoring equipment kept going wrong.

The clip on the baby's head was not registering the fetal heart, so another monitor was strapped round her abdomen.

> After five hours I was beginning to tire of riding the pain. Jo said, "Don't worry about the other people, just breathe, keep breathing, you're doing well, you've made it, well done!" . . . At the point where I was tiring a nurse did a vaginal exam and I was only five to six centimeters dilated! I thought another five hours of this is impossible, but Jo said to me, "You know it goes much quicker from now on."

Coping Alone

Felicia said it was a "marathon." She kept asking Jo for water, who put a small sponge soaked in icy water from the thermos in her mouth to suck. Her mouth became very dry because when she reached the end of the first stage most of her breathing was done through her mouth. Sometimes Jo could hardly get to the flask before another contraction came. "She also wiped my face with a warm washcloth. I especially liked to feel that on my cheeks and her warm hand on my arm through the contractions."

At last she began to want to push, and here Jo takes over again:

> I kept gently tipping her head down so that her chin was tucked in as she tended to throw her head back. There seemed to be no progress and the doctor came in ready to do a forceps delivery. Then as they got her feet into stirrups the baby's head rounded the corner and Felicia said she could feel it. Someone looked and said, "I can see the top of the head." I said to Felicia, "You're going to do it yourself after all." The doctor said, "I think I'm going to see a normal birth. I haven't seen one for years. See if you can break my run." I dashed down to see and saw a little dark mass and rushed up and told her I could see the baby's head.

Felicia pushed; the baby slid out and was given to her to hold immediately.

Black tendrils of hair damp from the womb, cheeks like a ripe peach, and huge eyes, violet-blue, looking straight up to her. She was plump and firm and amazingly hot, straight from a tropical uterine climate. The mother was laughing and crying at the same time. She drew the baby closer, holding her hungrily, devouring

.with her eyes the reality of this little person who stared at her quite calmly, as if to say: "So this is my mother!" Jo was crying, too. Her arm was around Felicia as she held the child. Their closeness was like petals touching, overlapping, folded in and curving over the baby.

A Chance to Grow

To have a baby when you are well over thirty is not just a case of "panic-breeding," a failure of nerve when faced with the shortness of life, the inadequacy of personal achievement, and the basic loneliness of every individual.

The birth of a child can be, and is for many women, an opening up of the new, an unfolding of love, not only for the baby, but perhaps for those from whom we have been guarding and protecting ourselves, and a step on the journey toward deeper understanding of ourselves and others. We can never possess our children. But through them, and with their help, we have a chance to grow as human beings.

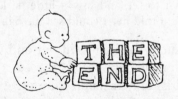

Notes

Chapter 2: Planning Ahead for Pregnancy

1 "Masculinization of the female fetus due to use of orally given progesterone," L. Wilkins, *Journal of American Medical Association* 172: 1028–32, 1960.

2 "Birth defects and oestrogen and progesterone in pregnancy," S. Harlap et al, *The Lancet* 1: 692–3, 1975; "Epidemiological problems associated with studies of the safety of oral contraceptives," D. Seigal and P. Corfman, *Journal of American Medical Association* 203: 950, 1968; "Oral contraception: potential hazards of hormone therapy during pregnancy," J. Robertson-Rintoul, *The Lancet* 2: 1315, 1974.

3 "Factors governing IUD performance," R. P. Bernard, *American Journal of Public Health* 61: 559–67, 1971.

4 "Possible prevention of neural-tube defects by preconceptual. vitamin supplement," R. W. Smithells, S. Shepherd et al, *The Lancet* 339–340, 16 February 1980.

5 "Double-blind randomized controlled trial of folate treatment before conception to prevent recurrence of neural-tube defects," K. M. Laurence, Nansi James et al, *British Medical Journal* 282: 1509–1511.

6 "Cigarette smoking in pregnancy and fetal hyperviscos-

ity." Peter C. Buchan, *British Medical Journal* 286: 1315, 1983.

7 "Smoking during pregnancy," B.B.K. Pirani, *Obstet. Gynecol: Survey* 33, 1, 1–13, 1978; *Smoking and Health. A Report of the Surgeon General* (U.S. Department of Health, Education and Welfare, 1979), Chapter 8; "Cigarette smoking in pregnancy." Leader in *British Medical Journal,* 28 August 1976.

8 "Sperm abnormalities and cigarette smoking," H. J. Evans et al, *The Lancet* 8221, Vol 1, 21 March 1981.

9 "The fetal alcohol syndrome," *Drug Abuse and Alcoholism Newsletter II:* 4, May 1978.

10 "Alcohol and advice to the pregnant woman," Griffith Edwards, *British Medical Journal* 286: 247, 1983.

11 Adapted from *Obstetrics,* Gordon Stirrat, Grant McIntyre, London, 1981.

12 "Hyperthermia as a possible teratogenic agent," David W. Smith et al, *Journal of Pediatrics* 92, 6, 878–883, June 1978; "Maternal hyperthermia as a possible cause of anencephaly," Peter Miller et al, *Lancet* I: 8063, 519–521, 1978.

13 "How does strenuous maternal exercise affect the fetus?" Susan L. Woodward, *Birth and the Family Journal* 8: I, 1981.

Chapter 3: Will the Baby Be All Right?

1 "Antenatal diagnosis of cytogenetic abnormalities," J. Simpson, *Seminars in Perinatology,* 4, 3, 168, 1980.

2 "Estimated rates of clinically significant cytogenetic abnormality (other than Down's syndrome) by one year maternal age intervals," E. B. Hook and D. K. Cross, *The American Journal of Human Genetics* 31: 136a, 1979.

3 "An antilactogenic effect of pyrodoxine," M. D. Foukas,

Notes

Journal of Obstetrics and Gynaecology of British Commonwealth 80: 718–20, 1973.

Chapter 4: Prenatal Care

1 "Maternal perception of fetal motoractivity," Keith Hertogs et al, *British Medical Journal* II: 6199, 1183–5, 1979; "Fetal activity and fetal wellbeing," J. F. Pearson and J. B. Weaver, *British Medical Journal* I: 1305–7, 1976; "Fetal movements," J. F. Pearson, *Nursing Mirror,* 21 April 1977; "Maternal perception of fetal movement and perinatal outcome," W. F. Rayburn et al, *Obstetrics and Gynecology,* 56,2: 161–5, 1980.
2 *An Interesting Condition: The Diary of a Pregnant Woman,* Abigail Lewis, Odhams, London, 1951.
3 "Twenty-four-hour studies of fetal respiratory movements and fetal body movements in normal and abnormal pregnancies," A. Roberts et al, *The Current Status of Fetal Heart Rate Monitoring and Ultrasound in Obstetrics* 209–20, R.C.O.G, London, 1977.

Chapter 5: Doctors

1 *Men Who Control Women's Health,* Diana Scully, Houghton Mifflin, Boston, 1980.
2 *Subject Women,* Ann Oakley, Robertson, Oxford, 1981.
3 *Some Women's Experiences of Induction,* Sheila Kitzinger, National Childbirth Trust, London, Second Edition, 1978.
4 *Maternal-Infant Bonding,* Marshall Klaus and John Kennell, Mosby, St. Louis, 1976.
5 *Practical Obstetric Problems,* Ian Donald, Lloyd-Luke, London, 1979. 5th edition, Harper & Row, New York, 1979.
6 Donald, ibid.
7 "The changing epidemiology of mortality and morbidity

in mothers and babies in recent years." Paper presented at a Study Group on Problems in Obstetrics organized by the Medical Information Unit of the Spastics Society. Tunbridge Wells, April 1975; "Induction of labour and perinatal mortality," R. H. Tipton and B. V. Lewis, *British Medical Journal* 1: 361, 1975.

8 Donald, op. cit.
9 "Induction and acceleration of labour in modern obstetric practice." Paper presented at a Study Group on Problems in Obstetrics organized by the Medical Information Unit of the Spastics Society. Tunbridge Wells, April, 1975.
10 See *Birth Rites, Birth Rights,* Judith Lumley and Jill Astbury, Sphere, Australia, 1980.
11 "Antecedents of handicap," Ross G. Mitchell, *Lancet* II 821:86–7, 1981.

Chapter 6: Life After the Baby Comes

1 In *Winter Trees,* Sylvia Plath, Faber, London, 1972. Harper & Row, New York, 1972.
2 *The Edible Woman,* Margaret Atwood, Virago, London, 1980. Warner Books, New York, 1983.

Chapter 7: Partners

1 *Maternal Care and Mental Health,* John Bowlby, London, World Health Organization, 1951; *Child Care and the Growth of Love,* John Bowlby, Penguin, London, 1953; *Attachment,* John Bowlby, Penguin, London, 1971. Basic Books, New York, 1969.
2 "The development of social attachments in infancy," H. R. Schaffer and P. E. Emerson, *Monographs of Social Research in Child Development,* 29, 3, 1–77, 1964.
3 *A World of Women,* Erica Bourguignon, Praeger, New York, 1980.
4 *The Speaking Tree: A Study of Indian Culture and So-*

ciety, Richard Lannoy, Oxford University Press, New York, 1971.

5 Sheila Kitzinger, unpublished research in Jamaica; *Women as Mothers,* Sheila Kitzinger, Fontana, 1978. Random House, New York, 1979.

6 "Depressive illness in general practice," A. M. W. Porter, *British Medical Journal* 28 March, 773–8, 1970.

7 *Feminine Personality and Conflict,* J. M. Bardwick et al, Wadsworth, Belmont, California, 1970.

8 *Subject Women,* Ann Oakley, Robertson, Oxford, 1981. Pantheon, New York, 1981.

9 *Biorhythms and Human Reproduction,* edited by Michel Ferin et al, Wiley, New York, 1974.

10 *Biological Rhythms in Psychiatry and Medicine,* G. G. Luce, U.S.P.H.C. 2088, U.S. Dept. of Health, Washington, D.C., 1970.

11 Ferin et al, op. cit.

12 "Emotional cycles in man," R. B. Hersey, *Journal of Mental Science* 77, 151–69, 1931.

13 Luce, op. cit.

14 *Sex Differences in Behavior,* H. Persky in R. C. Friedman et al, Wiley, New York, 1978.

15 *Parent-Infant Bonding,* second edition, Marshall H. Klaus and John H. Kennell, Mosby, St. Louis, 1982.

Chapter 9: Coping Alone

1 *Maternity Care in Ferment,* Maternity Center Association, New York, 1980.

Index

Index

Index

Index